ASTHMA

*Is Your Suffering
Really Necessary?*

ASTHMA

Is Your Suffering
Really Necessary?

WILLIAM W. FOX, MB, MRCS

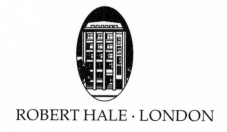

ROBERT HALE · LONDON

ISBN 0 7090 5705 9

Robert Hale Limited
Clerkenwell House
Clerkenwell Green
London EC1R 0HT

2   4   6   8   10   9   7   5   3   1

Photoset in North Wales by
Derek Doyle & Associates, Mold, Clwyd.
Printed in Great Britain by
St Edmundsbury Press Ltd, Bury St Edmunds, Suffolk.
Bound by WBC Book Manufacturers Limited,
Bridgend, Mid-Glamorgan.

Contents

Acknowledgements

I am deeply grateful to Dr Vernon Coleman and Dr David Freed, both of whom entrusted me to make use of their publications without let or hindrance.

This book is dedicated with everlasting love to my parents who taught me, by precept and practice, compassion for the poor and afflicted. Added to this was the imperative injunction never to demean those you are trying to help.

Preface

Health, Illness and Disease

In order to follow the main theme of this book, it is essential that you understand the meanings I attach to the words *health, illness,* and *disease*. The differences are crucial to that understanding. Always refresh your mind by re-reading these explanations if you are in any doubt; in particular illness and disease have often been treated as synonymous terms, even by doctors.

Health is a state of the body and mind that gives rise to no symptoms. Fortunate persons eat, live and sleep without any problems save those related to work, recreation and human relationships. In other words, such people are not conscious of their bodies except in so far as they are a source of pleasure. They are therefore referred to as healthy or normal.

Illness takes place when the body is attacked by external agents such as bacteria or viruses. During this phase the body's defences get to work and the offending agent is destroyed or ousted from the body. This process commonly takes place in the case of colds, influenza and all the childhood illnesses – measles, chickenpox, and so on. The illness, which is experienced as a high temperature, restlessness, coughing, running eyes or noses, is really the reaction of a healthy body to an invading organism, and often ends in complete recovery without the need for any drugs.

For those patients aged between six months and two years who are suffering from asthma in its very early stages the symptoms should be relatively mild. It is, at this stage, an illness, and so susceptible to a cure, if we do not intervene with drugs for whatever reason. If the illness persists and gets worse, it then becomes a disease.

Disease is a state of the body in which resistance has failed, either totally or partially, and abnormal conditions are established in its tissues. This situation can develop from the types of illness referred to above, when the body's resistance proves unsuccessful, or it may develop from other causes without such an obvious relationship. This is when clinical medicine should be used to establish what has gone wrong, why it went wrong, and what can be done to remedy or solve the problem. That is the true function of a doctor.

Because of the defects in their training, doctors are confused into treating illness in the same way as disease. The results are at best ineffectual, but more frequently doctors' treatment actually interferes with nature's normal reaction and produces problems that they do not understand. The same attitude to disease spills over into professional approaches to pregnancy and childbirth, to my mind the most beautiful examples of normality. Normality is a condition that doctors have never discussed and certainly not met in medical wards during their training. Being disease-orientated, they don't think of the millions that are born normally, but only of the very, very rare abnormal cases.

In my book, *Arthritis: Is Your Suffering Really*

Necessary? I referred to the invaluable aid I received from all the patients I interviewed. Their combined wisdom stood in marked contrast to the negative attitude of the medical profession. The remarkable success of that book surprised the publishers. But, as they can confirm, my belief in the intelligence of you, the public, was fully justified. It is for this reason that I am asking you to read this book.

The sixty-three years' experience I have had of the medical profession gives me very little hope that its practitioners will ever realize what an unholy mess they are making of health care. Only by informed pressure from the nation as a whole can we hope to break down their resistance and put a stop to so much disease, some of which they are, involuntarily, maintaining and creating. The terrible tragedy is that they do not consciously exploit the public, nor are they criminals; they genuinely believe they are efficient and honest. This kind of thinking is the most dangerous – and will change only as the result of a mental revolution.

Introduction

Let me first reassure my readers that I am fully aware of the anxiety, strain and misery, as well as the disappointed hopes, endured by parents and their children who suffer from asthma.

Add to this private pain the statistical tragedy of an ever-increasing number of deaths, now over 2,000 per year. Against such a background it would be heartless, if not criminal, to offer false hopes of improvement or even cure. Nevertheless I do take it upon myself to advance a controversial claim: namely, at least 50 per cent of sufferers can be greatly helped to become free of the constant use of drugs and the ever-present fear of death. The successes will be roughly in inverse ratio to the duration of treatment and severity of the disease in individual cases.

In order to achieve this goal it is essential that doctors and patients should fully understand the basic nature of the disease: how it starts; why it starts; how it progresses; and what factors determine its severity. All this will be described in full detail and in language intelligible to both the public and to those doctors prepared to move beyond the prejudices of their training.

It is crucially important to understand the natural

history of a disease before any form of treatment can be undertaken. Throughout my professional life I have followed this precept, and I believe it should be the right of every patient and the outlook of every doctor. I believe it is the lack of analysis in this area that accounts for the colossal and abject failure of orthodox treatment.

In order to place this view in context for the medical profession and the public let me now reproduce the introduction of a typescript I wrote around 1977 entitled *The Sickness of Medicine*. Although it is some years ago it is even more relevant now than it was then.

It is my belief that the vast majority of the population, including the doctors themselves, accept that the quality of medical services is as good as is possible in the light of available knowledge. Any failure to improve the health of those who suffer is therefore ascribed to lack of money, which limits research, numbers of hospital beds and other medical facilities. Moreover, a shortage of funds is said to exacerbate the great burden of overwork with which general practitioners allegedly have to cope.

What is implied in these assumptions is that if the profession were provided with everything that it thinks it needs, doctors would eliminate hospital waiting-lists, improve the health of the nation and enable most people to live longer.

The profession admits that a number of its members share the weakness of the rest of the population, such as drinking, fornicating, dishonesty and mental disability. The General Medical Council looks after all these problems. So, dear public, you can safely leave your health and your life in their hands – nothing is left to chance.

Associations of all kinds plan their activities on the basic assumptions I have just described. For example, the Migraine Society, the Arthritis Association, the National Back Pain Association, among others, all collect money in order to raise awareness and improve the condition of those who suffer and their families. Their unquestioning trust in the medical profession is shown by the presence of doctors on their committees. The Patients Association, on the other hand, seeks to protect its members from the admitted shortcomings of individual doctors. Nowhere is the question raised as to whether the quality of the doctors themselves is as good as it should be, taking into account the medical knowledge that is currently available. Mind you, there are still prima-facie cases of medical neglect that fail to achieve justice, but these do not often come to light because of the almost insuperable obstacles laypeople have to face in trying to amass evidence. It is extremely difficult to get doctors to testify against each other, partly because it is letting the side down, partly because it is always easier to look for extenuating circumstances for colleagues' errors of judgement and sometimes because they really don't know what they are talking about.

Moreover, the intrinsic value of doctors' services has been questioned by many thinkers and social workers of all kinds. A remarkable philosophical analysis has been made of their findings in a book called *Limits to Medicine, Medical Nemesis: The Exploitation of Health 1976* by Ivan Illich. The author was originally a monk before becoming a philosopher, writer and teacher of medieval history. Despite his remarkable command of the English language, he has a tendency to write very long and convoluted sentences, which required me to read and reread the text in order fully to comprehend all he had to say. For this reason, only a relatively small number of people will, I believe, be able to read and understand the basic truth of his argument. Sadly his style, difficult for the average reader, has diminished the impact of an otherwise important book.

I was greatly impressed by his ability to pinpoint the many fallacies of medical practice, but was equally delighted that such a powerful intellect was expressing what I had long known to be true. His message is crystal clear: the public is being over-medicalized. Ordinary people are made to believe that good health and long life can be determined by the self-appointed angels of God: doctors. Who can blame them for believing this, when the government, the establishment and the media are forever representing doctors as all-powerful and all-knowing? Illich by contrast asserts that the medical establishment has itself become a major threat to health. He places the blame for this shocking state of affairs on the fact that the baser instincts of humanity, such as greed, vanity and self interest, afflict doctors quite as much as other professionals. For this reason he can see no hope of any improvement except by transforming the whole attitude of the profession and at the same time educating the public.

Illich's book created quite a stir among those

doctors who heard about or read it. Some had no hesitation in denouncing him as a menace to their great and noble profession. There was one outstanding exception: Dr David Horrobin, a humane and exceptionally well-educated doctor. He spent much of his time treating the poor and sick in Africa and elsewhere. He was never very happy with the medical services in Great Britain and Africa and sought to improve them. His ability was recognized when he was appointed as clinical research professor in Canada some years ago.

In reply to Illich he published his *Medical Hubris* in 1977. In this book he accepts the facts on which Illich based his arguments but disputes his subsequent interpretations. Although he agrees that the medical establishment has become a major threat to health, he believes that this dangerous state of affairs can be ameliorated by ensuring we recruit a better type of medical student. By this he means students that have first been educated in the arts and humanities prior to starting their medical training.

Professor Ian Kennedy, an outstanding member of the legal profession, was honoured by the BBC in being invited to deliver the 1980 Reith Lectures on Radio 4. His subject was 'The Unmasking of Medicine'. He underlined much of what Illich had written and undoubtedly brought greater under-standing to a much larger audience. Unlike Illich he tends to regard the medical profession as misguided and not really conscious exploiters of disease. His analysis of medical practice has led him to believe that the public should cease to look upon doctors as real scientists, high priests or magicians and realize that they have the same limitations as all mortals. Would that the doctors themselves realize it!

Here we have three people of undoubted ability agreeing that there is something seriously wrong with the medical services delivered by doctors, irrespective of defects in organization and administration.

Illich sees no hope of transforming the attitude of the entire profession to his way of thinking. In addition, the goal of educating the public is feasible only if you can demonstrate that medical thinking and treatment are wrong and how, in practical terms, the lot of the patient can be improved. This is what concerns them, not abstract philosophical and political questions.

Transforming medical attitudes is a herculean task that is doomed to total failure unless you can amass detailed evidence to show that accepted thinking is wrong. The history of nearly all medical innovators clearly shows how unreceptive and pig-headed is the vast majority of the profession. Dr Horrobin believes that a better-educated student would in time produce a more rounded profession that would eradicate the failures of the past. In practice a delay of some twenty years would elapse before these students reached positions of authority and influence. Moreover, given that these students would be following the same format of education and training as now, I seriously doubt whether more than 5 per cent of students would mature into the type of doctor both he and I hope for.

Professor Kennedy contents himself with laying

out the problems for all to see and contemplate but, as far as I can follow, offers no practical solutions.

Whilst these three great minds are agreed on the gravity of the problems, I do not believe they have identified the factors that have led to this situation. That is why there is a divergence between them on how the problems are to be overcome. I would argue strongly that the basic failure and continuing menace of medicine are due entirely to the method of education in the medical schools and hospitals.

I am a product of that education and should be in a good position to evaluate it. When I entered general practice in 1931, my mind was crammed with all the 'wonderful' knowledge obtained at the bedside, in lecture theatres and from books. I really believed that soon I would be diagnosing and successfully treating large numbers of ailing patients. In fact I discovered that about 80 per cent of the patients I met in general practice had complaints that were never covered in hospital. What I had encountered as a student were tuberculosis, cancer, rare diseases of the nervous system, heart disease, gastric and duodenal ulcers, gall bladder disease, the occasional case of pneumonia and so on.

It is no wonder that in common with so many medical students I sometimes thought I was developing symptoms from one of the above. That is a measure of how strongly these diseases were drummed into us. Most GPs will never see more than one or two of these cases in any one year. This consciousness of major disease is inculcated into students' minds to such a great extent that by the time they enter general practice it becomes difficult for them to believe that their patients can be unwell unless they can recognize one of the diseases they were taught.

Because they did not realize it themselves, none of our teachers told us how comparatively rare these diseases are, nor did they tell us that we would be seeing patients with complaints that did not fit into this pattern of disease. So we were left totally unprepared to deal with these situations. That is the failure of medical education and the reason why it is responsible for so much bad diagnosis and treatment. It is also the reason why so many patients are subjected to endless expensive investigations – many of which are unpleasant and exhausting. The doctors are searching for evidence of diseases they can recognize in patients who have diseases they don't recognize.

To understand how this sorry state of affairs came about, you must know how the standard medical education is structured. During the first two years a great deal of time is spent teaching anatomy and physiology, in other words how the human body is constructed and how it functions. It is done very thoroughly – some would say too thoroughly, for much that is taught is soon forgotten because of its irrelevance to general practice. Anatomy in particular has been scaled down in recent years for that very reason. The demand for its revision came from practising doctors, not from the professors and lecturers in anatomy; it would never have occurred to them that they were over-teaching their very own subject. They had no experience of general practice and certainly would not consciously relate their discipline to living people with an illness. All the other subjects that comprise the rest of medical education are taught in a similar way. The teachers tend to be experts in a specialized field who know precious little of anything else. Now specialists can become very competent in diagnosing their diseases and treating them if there is a successful method available; unfortunately, this is not the case in some diseases. Consultants' preoccupation with their own narrow field lessens or even eliminates their interest in other illnesses or diseases, everything else can be left to other specialists! There is, therefore, an expert for every known disease or group of diseases, but none for any patient who cannot be diagnosed. However, the vast majority of patients do not have illnesses or diseases that fit snugly into these neat categories; they are therefore passed from one specialist to another, often being submitted to a series of futile investigations. It is this mass of patients that eventually have to be treated by the GPs, who know no more than the specialists. This signals the end of the line: a narrow quest has ended up in the alleviation of a meaningless bundle of symptoms by way of drugs, whose long-term use can have devastating effects on the patient.

It is in this way that doctors' critical and diagnostic faculties, their most important assets, and for which they have been trained, become blunted and wither.

A further defect in the system is that specialists might know masses of facts about their subject without having any real understanding of the disease itself. The outstanding examples are rheumatism and arthritis, with which my previous three books dealt in great detail. Young doctors who are appointed to the rheumatic departments and eventually become specialists in rheumatology have generally had no worthwhile experience in general practice. This might have taught them, as it taught me, that these diseases start long before X-rays show physical evidence of arthritis, which is the starting point for their diagnosis and study.

It is really like trying to solve a mystery story by reading only the second half of the book. You have missed all the clues in the first half, so that when further, corroborating evidence appears in the second half, it has no significance. It represents the difference between Sherlock Holmes and Peter Sellers's Inspector Clouseau, whose only hope was bumbling along until the truth popped up fortuitously.

Asthma is in the same category of diseases that are badly treated, and for the same reasons.

May I say that I was aware of these dangers more than thirty years ago, and in the early 1970s I tried very hard to get published *The Sickness of Medicine*, from which the above passage is taken. Needless to say, given its controversial nature, I failed to interest any medical publishers nor general non-fiction publishers. My final effort was with Robert Hale Ltd. I told my wife if they refused, I would give up and resign myself to a peaceful life looking after my patients. I had done exactly this several times before, but I always came back!

The refusal duly arrived. I kept my word and put the script away with the last one. About six months later, I got a telephone call from one of the directors at Robert Hale, who told me there had been a long discussion about my book before they decided not to publish, and he made it clear that he had been in favour. However, having read my chapter on asthma and hay fever, he was ringing to find out if I could help. He had a daughter aged twelve, who for the last five years had been suffering from severe asthma. The parents, while deeply distressed about the child, believed that she was being treated as efficiently as medical knowledge allowed. In all, they had been given three separate opinions; I was the fourth.

The girl was never well. Indeed she had missed so much of her education that the question of special schooling was under consideration, even though her parents knew she was mentally very bright. But she was only as tall as her sister, who was two years younger and she was unable to play games or go near a stable or farm. She was being treated for bronchitis and asthma with cortisone, courses of antibiotics, and more besides. The treatment I instituted was to stop all 'treatment', except for a little ephedrine and manipulation of the dorsal spine, because her chest was rigid after so many years of bad breathing. She soon improved and within one month there was no more asthma. Her chest expansion is now normal. She had developed rapidly, gaining weight and stature. In the following year she missed no school except for the odd day; there was no more talk of special school.

The director in question then went back to the boardroom at Robert Hale, and told them the story. He argued that since my treatment of asthma was effective,

I was likely to be right about the other subjects dealt with in the book. The company chairman still had strong doubts that a book dealing with so many different problems would sell. But in view of the compelling evidence he agreed that if I would write a book dealing solely with arthritis, the board would give it serious consideration. The book was finally published in 1981 (as *Arthritis: Is Your Suffering Really Necessary?*), and proved more successful than they ever expected. The book's good sales certainly got me a hearing by some of the more open-minded rheumatologists, but the red tape and financial constraints, before trials could be officially started, swallowed up eleven years of effort. In 1992 the problems were finally overcome, trials were initiated and are still ongoing – the results may be out in a year or so.

As I approach the twilight of my years, I am haunted by the spectre of all those children who could be saved from needless suffering and early death. To have lived so long and practised as a doctor for over sixty-five years is not enough – the lesson of studying patients' problems, without uncomprehending recourse to the prescription pad, must be learnt by all doctors.

All babies are beautiful: they create joy, happiness, hope and goodwill. By the age of five they display such intelligence that I often wonder why we do not, by now, have a nation of geniuses. As a nation we do very well, and generally we are still trying to improve everybody's lot. The work of politicians, religious leaders, educators, industrialists and trade unionists is in the public domain, there to be seen and evaluated. Discussion and free speech put continual pressure on these people to do the right thing. Medicine is the exception. It cannot be intelligently discussed by laypeople, because they know so little of the many subjects that doctors have to learn before they qualify. They know nothing of the relevance of teaching to the practice of medicine, for the results cannot be measured as they can in other spheres. In most trades or professions failure to satisfy clients or customers produces inevitable results – a loss of support and ultimately bankruptcy. In medicine this failure cannot be detected, from outside, by the patients, and is not recognized, inside, by the doctors. They are all waiting for the researchers, the laboratory technicians and the pharmaceutical firms to supply the wonder drugs that will solve all their problems. But you cannot solve a problem until you fully understand it, and this can be achieved only by grappling with it.

In my latest book on arthritis I have indicated the lines along which a better understanding of diseases will be achieved. My qualifications are simply a lifetime spent studying the early manifestations of the disease in childhood and beyond – in living, suffering human beings who taught me everything I know because I listened and examined. Look at any orthodox medical textbook on arthritis and you will see that the disease is not deemed to exist until there is evidence of joint damage and negative blood tests. How do the teachers of arthritis imagine it begins? Do they think it steals into the body overnight, producing visible arthritis in a joint the next day?

This century doctors have been overwhelmed with developments in medical science, starting with insulin for diabetes in 1920: antibiotics came in 1940; steroids in 1950; improved anaesthetics, making more and more operations possible; better X-rays and scanners; endless supplies of drugs to relieve and cure almost everything. This great march of progress was fuelled by all the diseases we could recognize and came about thanks to the diligence of nineteenth-century doctors. But what has happened to the 80 per cent of patients of whose conditions no clear diagnosis can be made? Look around and ask yourselves why, with so much medical progress, is ill-health so widespread? No matter how much money is spent on the National Health Service, it can never satisfy the endless demand for treatment. The answer is that the profession has little or no idea what causes the mass of symptoms of which patients complain. They cannot make a diagnosis, so they treat the symptoms, which is the very antithesis of good medicine. That is why at least an eighth of hospital beds are filled by patients suffering from drug poisoning – iatrogenic disease – caused by doctors' prescriptions. Countless thousands of patients are subjected to prolonged, sometimes painful, but always expensive investigations in order to try and match their symptoms to something the doctors know. When this rigmarole of referrals culminates in a failure to identify any known disease, patients are often advised to visit psychiatrists. Unaware that there may be an undetected physical cause for their patients' symptoms, psychiatrists search to discover a psychological cause – which often leads to a faulty diagnosis and a harmful prescription of antidepressants. All this is due to the fact that the research for a coherent understanding of patients' symptoms, gone into so painstakingly in the nineteenth century, has been abandoned. A massive and expensive 'scientific' superstructure masks an abyss of ignorance about the patients' true problems.

I hope this introduction will enable you to understand much more clearly the condition of asthma from its earliest appearance. I am confident that a very high percentage of you will be able to confirm most of the details I shall describe in the ensuing pages.

1   Prelude to Asthma

No successful treatment of any disease can be achieved
until the disease itself is fully understood. Why does it
start? What causes it? How does its behaviour vary?
What effect does it have on the patient, and how can
this be controlled? In order accurately to study this
natural history of the disease, it is important to
recognize the very earliest signs and symptoms. You
have to be very sure of these and not get them confused
with those allied to other diseases that are similar. More
importantly, you need to remember that some
symptoms are the natural reactions to disturbances in
the body and not due to disease at all.

To this end, it has been my philosophy to explain to
the patient as simply as possible what we know about
the disease, how it develops and what can currently be
done to control or cure it. Such an approach makes the
patient a more intelligent partner in the treatment
process. It is quite amazing the extent to which this
attitude removes fear from the minds of patients, how
gratefully they will accept any responsibility placed on
them by the doctor and how often they will be content
not to take drugs if so advised. Such a relationship
between doctor and patient can be established only if
the doctor is aware in each case of the potential

limitations of diagnosis and treatment.

I have never been afraid to tell patients that I did not understand their cases because a diagnosis could not be made in terms of accepted medical teaching. But I always tried. It was in this way that I pieced together the evidence to construct a more coherent picture of the truth.

As asthma often begins in the early weeks or months of a baby's life, let us first consider the problems which may beset the new arrival. There are two which are basic to the understanding of asthma: *teething* and *infection*.

Teething

Between six to nine months of age the milk teeth start to arrive and continue forming until two years old or a little longer. The teething process is frequently heralded by restlessness, bad temper, crying and slobbering at the mouth. The child oftens stuffs his hand into the mouth or rubs his face, refuses to take food and gets feverish – temperatures of 30°C plus are quite common. Sometimes the chest gets wheezy. The number and severity of these symptoms vary with the difficulty or ease with which the tooth breaks through the gum. The duration of the symptoms depends on how long the tooth takes to makes its appearance. Immediately it happens, all the symptoms disappear and the child very quickly returns to its normal happy self.

There is no obvious reason why children should vary so much in their reaction to cutting a tooth, but the important point to remember is that it is not a disease and does not require medical treatment in the form of drugs. I can understand why parents get anxious under these circumstances. There are, however, two important aspects that they can easily check for themselves. If the baby's crying is strong and lusty and you can hardly hold him or her in your arms because of so much energetic movement, the baby is unlikely to have any serious ailment. A very sick child does not cry loudly but moans rather softly; it is too ill to throw itself about and lies restlessly in your arms or the cot. Fortunately, babies are rarely seriously ill, meaning that parents do not tend to see this latter type of case. Therefore it is difficult for them to recognize the difference and thus not to be alarmed. It is not surprising that they will ask the doctor's advice. I do not know how many doctors are aware of this important difference in the significance of symptoms because I have not seen it mentioned in any recent medical textbooks.

In my early days in general practice there were no antibiotics or tranquillizers. There was no method of 'treating' the wide variety of symptoms encountered, beyond a little aspirin. I therefore had no alternative but to witness how they developed and apply the art and skills of examination and observation so meticulously taught to me as a student. These skills were used in hospital to help in the diagnosis of diseases, such as cancer and diabetes, that were then recognizable. Our professors were able to identify them precisely because an earlier generation of doctors had pinpointed the clinical signs and symptoms by their own observations of the disease before they knew what they were. That is exactly what I was anxious to do.

Now let us go back to babies and consider two signs that occur in many of their teething episodes. First the child keeps rubbing or hitting its ear, implying that the pain is there. Sometimes one would see a congestion of the ear-drum, suggesting the onset of an acute inflammation. There was nothing I could do but wait and explain the problem to the parents. Invariably the condition got better within a day or so, usually coinciding with the eruption of a tooth. I then realized that the congestion and pain in the ear were just part of the teething story and was therefore able to reassure the parents. Teething in children is inevitable and common; middle-ear disease is extremely rare and probably never occurs at this age and in these circumstances. The point of this example is that when using diagnostic skills it is every bit as important to recognize when disease is absent as when it is present.

I recently read an article in an American health magazine by two child specialists. They referred to a relatively high number of babies who have suffered attacks of middle-ear disease, some of whom having had as many as three such attacks in the first eighteen months of life. They then stressed the importance of giving antibiotics immediately and of monitoring the child closely to make sure improvement occurs within thirty-six hours. A lack of progress would mean that a change of antibiotic was mandatory.

There can be very few doctors practising today who started their careers before the age of the antibiotic about forty years ago. I suppose there were other doctors like myself who learned from experience that this 'ear inflammation' was not serious and soon got better without treatment. There was no way that anyone could have communicated this knowledge to our professors and teachers, much less persuaded them that it was true. To achieve this one would have had to produce evidence from a large sample – an impossible task for a GP. Even as a full-time project, proof would have been virtually impossible with the rudimentary technology available then. But even assuming these practical obstacles could have been removed, a lowly GP would have been extremely fortunate to interest the *British Medical Journal* or the *Lancet*, the only two medical journals with significant circulation figures, in publication within their hallowed pages.

So we are in a position where the specialists, totally unaware of the cause of this relatively harmless condition, pontificate on its seriousness and the necessity for close supervision and treatment.

By the 1990s otitis media had become so prevalent that ear specialists began to take a greter interest in this problem. They described the details of the early signs of inflammation of the eardrum and the general symptoms of apparent infection of the upper respiratory tract. Being specialists they did not see and therefore omitted all the details of the baby's behaviour which I have described. They also reported that the peak of these illnesses are first reached by the age of two and that 80 per cent of all these cases completely recover within three days without any treatment! Isn't that exactly what I have written excepting that I have given a fuller clinical picture of the problem and a sensible explanation of the symptoms and the outcome?

I must add that in all my years of practice I saw only one child of five who had what they now call glue ear. I performed a paracentesis (making a slight cut in the eardrum) and he quickly lost his pain and soon recovered. I suspect that in the case of the 20 per cent of children who require further treatment, the antibiotics they had been given may have contributed to their problems.

There must be countless thousands of parents who have given their babies antibiotics in these circumstances, in the belief that tragedies were being averted.

The second symptom is wheezing in the chest. This seems almost always to be called bronchitis, a diagnosis that, in a well nourished society like ours, I am absolutely sure is wrong in the vast majority of cases. It is in fact an allergic reaction of the lungs in susceptible babies during a teething episode. It will be fully discussed later. For the moment, you can assume that it is no more serious than the 'ear disease' just described and will disappear when the tooth erupts.

In both these cases, all those doctors who do not recognize the significance of the symptoms are quite likely to think the child is developing acute ear disease, bronchitis or pneumonia and immediately prescribe an antibiotic. When the child recovers in a day or so everybody (including the doctor) thinks, How marvellous! The child has been rescued from middle-ear disease, bronchitis, pneumonia or even death. This is the way in which laypeople become dependent on the medical profession and antibiotics – a perfect illustration of Illich's suspicions (see Introduction), but which without medical knowledge he was unable to explain.

From such a perspective it is a short step to prescribing an antibiotic for any child with a feverish condition, just in case it might become serious. This problem will be dealt with when I discuss infectious disease. The correct treatment for the so-called ear infection is reassurance for the parents and a little loving for the baby, with the addition of a teething ring and maybe a tiny dose of paracetamol. The same treatment is equally appropriate for the 'bronchitis' types. If the wheezing is severe a little ephedrine can be administered, but the effects will be minimal.

After studying this phenomenon for some time, I have become convinced that if you allow the illness to take its own course the baby will develop a natural tolerance to the allergy's source. As you will see, no child under my care ever failed to come through these wheezy asthmatic episodes and finally achieve their own cure. So why has there been such a dramatic increase in the deaths linked to a disease that throughout its history was never a killer? This problem will be further discussed in Chapter 3 alongside a paper written by Dr David L.J. Freed, an allergist who has worked with me for many years and was my joint author on a recent book, *Understanding Arthritis*.

The picture I sketched for you of a baby in the throes of teething, with a high temperature, wheezing, coughing, screaming and restless banging its head or ears with its tiny hands can be very frightening. The GP is summoned and the wonder drug – an antibiotic – is prescribed. As one GP put it in a BBC interview, 'I give an antibiotic first and try to make a diagnosis later if the child does not improve.' As you now know, the baby most often recovers without treatment. Alas, present-day GPs think they have cured the sickness – perhaps even saved the child's life.

What are the consequences? Not only did the antibiotic do no good, its presence in the immune system of the child must have a confusing effect. When this form of treatment persists for every similar episode, the damage becomes cumulative. Meanwhile allergic reactions to some of these antibiotics can serve to aggravate asthma.

Infectious Diseases
Scientific medicine, by way of vaccination, has made quite remarkable progress in eradicating or minimizing many diseases such as smallpox, polio, measles and

whooping cough. Where this has not been possible antibiotics have been provided to kill the germs in diseases like pneumonia, meningitis and some forms of bowel inflammation.

Despite all this progress children still get fevers, colds, coughs and sore throats. All of these are caused by germs invading the mucous membrane, which is the lining of the nose, throat and bronchial tubes leading to the lungs. The adenoids behind the nose and the tonsils in the throat are the frontline barriers against these attacks and are essential for the proper defence of the body. The adenoids and tonsils contain lymphatic tissue in which the germs get trapped. This tissue has the special functions of alerting the body's defences to attack and destroying these invading organisms. This is exactly how the body becomes accustomed to fighting disease, a form of learning that develops the natural immunity we need to survive. When we give a vaccine to a healthy child, what we are doing is educating the body to resist the invasion of a laboratory-grown germ that has been rendered much less harmful than it would be in its natural state. The effect of this is to shorten the learning period by possibly a generation or two.

A vaccine can be effective only when the germ has been identified and isolated. Where this has not been achieved, we must witness children doing their own fighting, which in the vast majority of cases ends in recovery. Once you understand this rather simple problem, the urgency and anxiety that many parents feel when their child is ill should rather be turned to wonderment at the remarkable resilience that nature has bestowed on the human race. The child needs nothing but parental love and care, perhaps augmented by a simple syrup for the cough.

There are a few children who might not have the good fortune to recover as quickly as most, but given a day or so they probably will. If they do not, there is still ample time to prescribe an antibiotic, if it is suitable. Bear in mind that the extra day or so before it is used is not wasted – far from it: the body is learning how to cope more effectively with the next attack.

The success of my approach has been achieved by educating my patients exactly as described in the text.

In order to widen and apply this knowledge it is essential that all GPs are capable of making these distinctions in diagnosis. So far they show no signs of this ability, judging by the widespread use of antibiotics and the pragmatic approach of their teachers.

Let me give you an example. Many years ago a patient of mine in her early twenties, married and went to live near St Albans. One day she developed a severe acute headache with marked stiffness of the neck. The GP was called and he diagnosed possible meningitis. A consultant was called in and confirmed such a possibility. The girl's mother was present. Due to the education I had given her during her daughter's childhood, she actually challenged the diagnosis and refused to allow her daughter to be taken to hospital unless I confirmed the diagnosis.

Accordingly, she phoned and gave me all the details. I explained to her the impossibility of my getting to St Albans until very late that day and only then if the GP agreed. Also, I was not prepared to advise her to bring her daughter to London which she asked me to do. I emphasized the risk of delayed treatment if it was meningitis.

Judge my surprise when she arrived at my consulting rooms a couple of hours later. I saw her immediately. To my astonishment, the young lady, apart from the severe headache and stiff neck did not present a clinical picture of an acute disease remotely resembling meningitis.

On examination I discovered a rheumatic patch in the neck which was the sole cause of her symptoms. A suitable injection was given (details are available in any of my books) and she got up free of her headache and stiffness.

The inferences to be deduced from this story are:

(1) Doctors are not well trained in differential diagnosis. This ignorance of the rheumatic patch will become clear to you in the final chapter.
(2) A well educated layperson (who knew about the rheumatic patch) was able to make a judgement that her daughter probably did not have meningitis – as she said to me 'my daughter did not seem ill enough for such a diagnosis'.

Of course doctors will dismiss this story as 'anecdotal', which means it cannot have any real value unless confirmed by many other cases. I would remind them that meningitis is very rare. In fact, I have never seen a case in the whole of my professional life which spans over sixty years. Furthermore, the wrong diagnosis will hardly ever come to light because as I have explained, natural recovery is not recognized – the antibiotic is the cure all!

If you have followed my analysis, you should understand that none of these common conditions, however severe, constitutes disease. Most such symptoms are the expression of the body's healthy reactions to an invading germ. The 'illness' will soon be over and the child will be all the healthier for the experience.

Furthermore, most of these illnesses are caused by viruses, which cannot as yet be destroyed by antibiotics. They are quite different from the bigger germs – bacteria – which can.

I do believe that the wholesale removal of tonsils and adenoids, which was common practice in my early days, has been dramatically curtailed. Nevertheless, a word of caution and advice can do no harm. The snoring, difficulty in breathing and consequent apparent lack of appetite that many children experience is brought about by the pad of adenoids situated behind the nose. Because of the upright position that humans have adopted, the adenoids, especially when swollen by infection, tend to aggravate the nasal blockage. If the problem is persistent, it is justifiable to scrape the central part away in order to leave the nasal passage free. It is a very minor procedure that I did for several children in their own homes with a minimum of fuss and expense. I did it because I knew if I sent them to a hospital the tonsils and adenoids would be removed as a matter of routine, even though the tonsils were still doing an important job in frontline defence. The only justification for the removal of tonsils is when they are so diseased by repeated infection that they can no longer perform their function adequately.

There are two other kinds of infection I would like to tell you about. First, influenza. This is a virus infection that occurs in epidemics; some of the viruses have been identified and vaccines have been used for many years. Their success in reducing the number of people affected is accepted, as are their great value in protecting older people who have not developed a natural resistance. A perfect example is myself. I suffered almost yearly attacks of influenza, which greatly undermined my health and strength. Since the advent of the vaccine, I have enjoyed a much higher standard of health and stamina. There are, however, new strains of viruses causing exactly the same symptoms as influenza, for which vaccines have not yet been developed, or which are not considered too serious, because by and large natural immunity is gradually learning to overcome them.

The second problem concerns colds. Over the years researchers have laboured to identify a number of different viruses as possible causes. However, they have not been able to reproduce the 'cold' effectively in people who allowed the viruses to be installed in their noses in order to establish a true causal relationship.

Now let me put the cold, or coryza, problems in simple terms that any layperson can understand. Germs and viruses are everywhere, looking for the right conditions in which to breed; the human body happens to be an effective hunting ground for some of them. They enter the nasal passages and immediately start to invade the mucous membrane; if they succeed they can penetrate the defences and get into the body cells. These cells may be nerve, liver, kidney, lung or connective tissue. Once established, these viruses can cause people to become ill with various diseases, some of which we can recognize as influenza, hepatitis, nephritis, sleeping sickness and (I believe but cannot prove) multiple sclerosis.

If, however, the body reacts against the virus, a streaming cold is the result; you feel rotten for a few days, then all is well. In other words, you have won the fight against the invader and developed an immunity to the virus. This development of resistance is a key facet of the survival of the fittest, and should be welcomed by the profession. It exactly fits my description of an illness, as opposed to a disease.

During the first five to six years of a child's life, the vast majority of its 'illnesses' are likely to be viral infections or linked to teething. In these cases the widespread use of antibiotics cannot possibly be justified on medical grounds. Apart from doing untold harm to many children, it costs millions of pounds – money that could be used for real scientific benefit elsewhere in the system.

To support these views, here are the details of two clinical experiments carried out over a number of years. The first concerns my daughter and her young children. They were living about 200 miles away when the following incidents took place. When the children fell ill, my daughter quite reasonably called out her GP to ensure that no serious condition was developing. Needless to say, every consultation resulted in a prescription for an antibiotic. This was followed by a phone call from my daughter, who had been thoroughly educated in my views on the matter. 'Guess what?' she would say, and my reply would be 'Another antibiotic! You know what to do.' 'Sure,' came the reply. 'Tear it up and save the National Health Service a lot of money.' These children never had an antibiotic – how many parents can say that?

The second experiment was even more illuminating. Again the mother (whom I shall call Mary) had two children, who I had looked after since birth. My views on teething, illness and antibiotics were carefully explained to her. After two teething episodes accompanied by very high temperatures in the first baby, she had the factual proof of my advice and the confidence to cope with future episodes. After that, at my request, she phoned to report further episodes and, subsequently, the children's complete recovery without any treatment.

When the children began to attend nursery school, more frequent and closer contact with other children created the opportunity for infections to spread. The most frequent were colds, chicken pox and German measles, none of which could possibly be affected by antibiotics.

Mary, who was now actively engaged in collecting evidence for me, questioned the parents of other children at the same school and found that antibiotics were invariably prescribed. On one particular occasion there was an outbreak of diarrhoea and vomiting at the school, probably due to tainted food. All the children were kept at home for a few days. Once again they were all given antibiotics by their doctors. Only the two under my care were given nothing: they were back at school within two days; many of the others took four to five days before returning to school.

I could add that I educated a considerable number of my patients to realize the folly of indiscriminate use of antibiotics and I trust my beliefs will be carried through to the next generation. A small but ever-growing number of thoughtful people now add their voices to the criticisms of conventional methods of treatment. Armed wth this knowledge, we can now consider the problem of asthma, from the earliest point of its onset through to its development and outcome.

2 Asthma and Hay Fever

Asthma is so characteristic a disease that it should present no real problem in diagnosis. The symptoms are wheeziness in the chest accompanied by an irritating cough with very little phlegm. The child's breathing becomes shorter and shorter, and the colour of the face changes from pale to red; in the more severe cases it can darken to a bluish hue. This striking facial colour combined with the child's gasping for air is a frightening picture, so it is little wonder that parents get anxious and concerned.

The illness is considered to be allergic in character. This means that all the symptoms described above are caused by the body's reaction to a substance with which it is not fully equipped to deal. This substance acts like an irritant and can enter the body mainly in two ways. First through the mucous membrane, that is the lining of the nose, throat or bronchial tubes and lungs. It can be a germ or virus, or pollen from flowers, trees, shrubs and plants. It is present in many forms of house dust, plastics, paint, newsprint and domestic pets of all kinds.

Secondly, it can be ingested through the mouth in the form of food and drink. It is often found in proteins: cows' milk, eggs, cheese and strawberries are a few examples. In addition we have to remember that in modern food production and processing a large variety of chemicals are used, some of which may be causing this kind of allergy. This category also includes drugs prescribed by doctors for other reasons. It may very well be that some of these chemicals are a contributing factor to the increasing number of asthma cases occurring in this and many other countries. Unfortunately there are no reliable statistics, because asthma, on account of its rarity, has never been a notifiable disease like, for example, diphtheria, the incidence of which has been carefully monitored every year since records were kept. The fact that the number of deaths was also recorded annually meant that it became a simple matter to determine the natural behaviour of the disease and the effect of medical treatment. In the case of asthma the problem has been compounded by the confusion in diagnosis between bronchitis and asthma, which has also given rise to much uncertainty about the true figures.

According to the Asthma Research Council, in the 1970s the number of people suffering the condition was known to be one million. However, some experts put the figure at closer to two million and rising. If we take this more realistic estimate and divide it by the approximate 30,000 doctors in general practice, we get an average of seventy cases for each GP. During my first twenty-five years as a GP, from 1931 to 1956, the maximum number of asthma cases I treated in any one year was five. I would say that the average number for this period would be two per annum and certainly not more than three. The Asthma Research Council figures represent a seventeen-fold increase on my maximum. I will later go on to discuss my high success rate in treating this disease, which will account for my own figures being so low. Allowing for this, I would suggest the increase in asthma over the last twenty years may well be in the order of 600 to 800 per cent.

In May 1979 the US Department of Health, Education and Welfare published a comprehensive report entitled 'Asthma and the Other Allergic Diseases'. They estimated the number of asthmatic cases to be 8.9 million out of a population of 235 million. Figures from Australia and New Zealand show the same trend. On an equivalent ratio, two million asthmatics would be a reasonable postulation for the 50 million people living in Britain. They, like us, have no reliable figures for previous years, but they were able to produce statistics covering the years 1969–1975, which showed the relative number of asthmatics per 1,000 of the population who presented themselves for treatment and/or sickness certificates. Here are the figures:

Year	Percentage of asthmatics
1969	8.1
1971	9.1
1972	8.7
1973	9.9
1974	11.6
1975	11.8

(1970 is not included because it did not appear in the report)

This indicates an increase of 47 per cent in seven years. While the report does not cover the previous nine years from 1960 – roughly the period when, I believe, the real increase began – it does not need much imagination to see that this half-fold increase could by 1980 easily equal the estimated 600 to 800 per cent rise that I projected from my experience.

The former Soviet Union published in English a handbook entitled 'Health Care in 1979'. They had by far the longest-running health service in the world, and therefore had no difficulty in providing statistics on any aspect of illness. Let me quote verbatim from the introduction:

> The advances in chemistry have meant not only an increase in soil fertility, the development of synthetic materials and all-purpose plastics which have revolutionized our living conditions, but also *a dramatic increase in allergic conditions in all their forms from coryza to asthma* [my italics]

The fact that the dramatic increase in asthma in the former Soviet Union, the United States and Great Britain did not occur in the developing countries of Africa and South America where antibiotics were not easily available, is important circumstantial grounds for arguing that antibiotics, freely available in the richer countries, could be the cause of the increase in asthma.

I have divided my study of asthma into two distinct periods, the first being before 1960, which is when I believe the number of cases began to increase, and the second being after this date. The reason for this apparently arbitrary decision will become clear later on.

I do not recall seeing more than a single case of asthma as a medical student either in the wards or the outpatients' department, so it is unlikely to have been very prevalent. One of the early cases I saw was a baby I had delivered in my own practice in 1931. I diagnosed the illness as a mild case of asthma that occurred when the baby was cutting a tooth. The face was deep red, breathing was short and I could hear wheezing in the chest even without a stethoscope. The child also had a temperature of 39°C. I remember thinking at the time how easily this case might be mistaken for acute bronchitis. In those days the GP's only option was to give the baby a harmless cough mixture – there were no antibiotics or sprays – and wait. Within a day or so, all the symptoms disappeared as soon as the tooth had come through – the baby was normal. It was definitely a mild asthma attack, for bronchitis would have lasted much longer. I explained this to the parents and said that the attacks were likely to recur with further teething episodes. In those days there was no question of doing allergy tests on a baby. We just took the sensible precautions of keeping wool, dust, and so on out of harm's way. A further attack did develop with teething episodes, but they always got better very quickly without treatment. In other words, I had reassured the parents, so they were not afraid of attacks and the baby gradually developed his own immunity. By the time his last tooth was cut the attacks had disappeared and for the six years he was under my care he remained totally free of asthma.

I was dealing with the child's first attack. The parents had not been subjected to the strain and anxiety of a child who had repeated bouts and they therefore had no idea how disturbing and frightening it could be. So it was no problem for them to be confident, cheerful and unafraid, creating in turn an atmosphere for the child where fear was absent. This is truly the best medication in the world, providing the doctor understands the natural behaviour of the illness and has confidence in the body's ability to develop its own immunity in time.

The next sensible procedure I adopted was to explain to parents that when the second or subsequent attack came along, it would be better if I did not appear, because the child would soon learn to associate the need for a doctor with each attack, and thus a subconscious dependence would begin to form. Asthma, without doubt, has its psychological aspects. They were always welcome to telephone me either when an attack started or any other time if they were worried. The arrangement worked perfectly: it saved the parents a lot of fees (I was a private doctor for there was no NHS), me a lot of time, and the children would eventually recover to complete health.

There was another aspect of the psychological problem which may occur only when the child has become a chronic asthmatic and has learned to exploit the situation either consciously or subconsciously.

These two aspects of the psychological problem in the so-called causation of asthma were all that mattered before 1960. How this has changed in the last three decades will be explained later.

What I want to impress on you now is that of the over seventy cases of childhood asthma that I looked after during my years in general practice, not one had any different treatment than what I have just outlined. I would occasionally administer a small dose of ephedrine to relax a severe bronchial spasm, but that was all. It should also be remembered that of all the other known asthma cases in the country, about 30 per cent developed their own immunity by the time of adolescence. Many of these became progressively desensitized and took steps to avoid the natural irritants I mentioned before. Given many of these children improved without my help, why was I so sure that my approach was right? After qualifying as a doctor I saw a few cases during my first two years as a houseman in hospital and as a locum for other GPs. The outstanding feature was the parents' anxiety and fear for the health and sometimes life, of their children. I believe this fraught emotional state was bound to affect the child and so aggravate the condition.

Who was responsible for this state of affairs? It could only be the doctors, who understood so little of the condition that they were unable to reassure the parents. These children were all four or five years old and were suffering from full-blown asthma. Why had the condition been allowed to develop to this chronic and frightening stage? All I could think of was that the very early attacks during the teething period were not recognized as early asthma but were called acute bronchitis and treated with ineffectual but harmless cough mixtures. The asthma attack would come to an end with the eruption of the tooth and all would be well until the next attack of 'bronchitis'. These episodes would be repeated at irregular intervals up to the end of the teething period (two to two-and-a-half years old). By then it should surely have been recognized as asthma and become a disease and not an illness.

Because this situation was neither understood nor taught in hospitals, the diagnosis depended on the imagination of young and inexperienced doctors. In the sequence of events you can see how the words bronchitis, bronchitis and asthma, bronchial asthma and finally asthma formed a chain to cover up medical confusion and uncertainty. All this stemmed from the basic fact that the specialists who taught students about asthma had probably never seen a baby in the teething stage with a wheezy chest and therefore had no idea about the link between the two, or if they had, they could not recognize it.

Scientific investigation and treatment began only when asthma was established as an identifiable, textbook disease. Those of you who have read my book *Arthritis: Is Your Suffering Really Necessary?* will notice the same basic fault. Diagnosis and study only began when arthritis could be demonstrated.

Against the background of my success in discouraging asthma to develop in any of my own cases, let us now consider some patients of mine in whom the condition was fully established and diagnosis was a straightforward issue. Their stories will illustrate the points I have already made.

As District Medical Officer I was responsible for the health of those people in the Darwen area who were living on income support. During this time, I was consulted by a widowed mother regarding her only child, a boy of ten years, who was suffering from severe asthma. In a case of this type I needed to make some visits to the family home to judge their relationship and the cleanliness of the rooms as well as to discuss matters of nutrition. I concluded that life at home was fraught with psychological disturbance – in particular, the mother's anxiety over her child was actually aggravating the symptoms. I explained this to her – and the fact that the boy knew instinctively how to get his own way about food, spending money or getting time off school: all he needed to do was to 'throw' an attack of asthma. His mother would then smother him with love and send for the doctor.

Unfortunately, she was not bright enough to co-operate and all my efforts were doomed to failure.

Every time he had an attack he turned very blue and his mother became certain he would die if the doctor did not come at once. To convince her of the psychological basis of the condition, I even resorted to giving the child injections of water instead of adrenaline. He always recovered from the attacks.

One night she rang my doorbell at 2.30 a.m. I refused to go with her and threatened to call the police if she did not desist from disturbing me. I went to see the boy later that morning – he was fully recovered. Shortly after this I left Darwen for London, so I do not know what became of this unhappy mother and child. What I had proved was that the boy could recover without treatment and that his mother's anxiety and short-sighted response were the real reasons for the asthma continuing.

The next example concerns three cousins, only one of whom was under my care. The first one was born into a wealthy family in London. He apparently had the benefit of all that money could buy: the leading specialists, nurses, devoted parents. This mother and father went to the lengths of buying a second house in Bournemouth, as the fresh air of the seaside, as well as the town's pine trees, were recommended by one of the doctors as being good for asthma. Nevertheless the boy remained a chronic asthmatic until after the death of both his parents. When I met him in the late 1970s he told me he had steadily improved since being on his own. His mother's distraught response to his illness was drummed into him over the years, and he had become brainwashed into being an invalid.

Cousin number two had much the same history, the main difference being that his mother died before World War II, when he was about sixteen years old. By the time the war started he was given a completely clean bill of health and became a bomber pilot! Neither of these cases was under my care, although I knew them. What is significant is the rapid improvement that took place after the death of the mothers. Sadly, the parents in question were the vehicles for the emotional anxiety that so adversely affects the asthmatic state. You will realize that I do not blame them; their anxiety was exacerbated by the failure of the medical attendants to understand this important aspect of the illness.

Cousin number three was some years younger than the other two. His story was similar to the first cousin who lived in London. When the boy was five years old, his parents were advised to move from Manchester to St Annes on Sea in Lancashire. This they did, but the attacks continued exactly as before. Knowing how asthma had ruined the other cousins' youth, the parents were very anxious and in desperation asked me if I could help. Despite being based some thirty miles away in Darwen, I agreed to look after him. I carefully explained my views about anxiety and environmental effect on the sufferer. All the mollycoddling and medicines were stopped (bar a small dose of ephedrine), and when an attack came on, I insisted on him going into the garden instead of to bed. In less than one month his asthma disappeared for good. He is now sixty-one, and lives in Australia. He makes a point of visiting me whenever he comes to Europe. I believe this has something to do with the memories of his asthmatic childhood and his complete freedom after I treated him.

Finally let me describe one of the first cases I encountered after moving to London: an 8-year old boy who suffered repeated attacks of asthma. Again, his wealthy parents had sought the best advice, but to no avail. When I first saw the child, parental anxiety was, as usual, palpable. I discovered two other factors, however, on my meticulous routine examination: one was the fixity of the chest wall, so that even if he could breathe properly his chest could not expand; the second was a very marked inability to breathe through his nose, particularly when he was eating. I thought this was due to what is called 'mal-occlusion' – a bad fit between the upper and lower jaws that gives rise to irregular teeth, inefficient chewing and poor intake of air through the nostrils. I was able to manipulate the bones of the chest (that is, the dorsal spine and the ribs), which allowed his lungs to expand more efficiently: almost at once his breathing became deeper and more normal. The condition of the nose and mouth slowly but surely improved with the aid of a mouth splint made by an orthodontist. Otherwise the treatment was exactly the same as ever, and so was the cure. The boy in question is now fifty-three, has very regular teeth, no breathing problems and only distant memories of asthma.

All these cases occurred before 1960. I earlier said I would explain the significance of this demarcation. Some twelve years after the establishment of the National Health Service, by 1960 everybody could have a doctor whenever required, and each doctor was free to prescribe any pill in their armoury without fear of hurting their patients financially. Surely health would improve. In the past the psychological aspects of asthma loomed large because the disease did not pose any threat of death: it was relatively easy to manage with small doses of ephedrine, or adrenaline for those rare acute episodes. The intensity of the attacks was never cumulative and quite clearly self-limiting – indeed these bouts of breathlessness are clearly nature's way of coping with the poison (allergy). The improvement and cure by nature's own efforts started in a few cases within a year or two and rose to about 30 per cent of all cases by the age of puberty.

No doubt many of those who recovered in later years would have been freed from the condition earlier if the element of fear had been understood by the specialists. The remainder generally lived into their seventies; though they had to cope with a disability, they hardly ever became invalids.

Whatever happened to asthma? Instead of diminishing, the numbers began to rise and deaths from asthma reached 1,000 in 1978. By 1981 the annual figure was up to 1,500. In a few years' time the statistic was 2,000 – and it is still increasing. This fact alone surely confirms my belief that the state of asthma treatment is deplorable, and demands an early investigation into the whole problem of diagnosis and treatment.

I have already indicated that the sharpness of the increase in numbers of cases can in part be accounted for by the chemicals used in food manufacture and processing. The allergy could also be explained by hormones in animal feed, which we later consume in meat. The widespread use of plastics has also been suggested as a cause by Russian scientists. Far more important, in my view, is the widespread use of antibiotics in the treatment of children's ailments.

There cannot be many doctors in practice today who have had any experience of the pre-antibiotic era. As explained in 'Teething' I learned to distinguish between real illness and the teething syndrome. As this has not been taught to the students when they go into General Practice these conditions are generally assumed to be serious and an antibiotic is prescribed. Only in the last few years have government circulars gone to GPs asking them to be more circumspect in prescribing these antibiotics, not because they suspected any harm but because they were expensive and wasteful. As there has been no remarkable improvement in the death rate of children over the last thirty years, the antibiotics can claim no success in this field and their widespread use must be suspect.

Let us consider how an antibiotic works. A precise, scientifically approved drug for killing known species of germs that make people ill, it works by direct action on the germs in the patient's body. The body, in most cases, is well able to take care of itself, because it has an innate mechanism for destroying the invading germ if given sufficient time. This is the period when both the patient is ill – for perhaps two to three days, or even up to three weeks and when the body is learning how to combat the disease by developing its own immunity. If you interpose an antibiotic during this stage, you interfere with the body's normal reaction and almost certainly cause confusion to the orderly behaviour of the immune system.

The only time an antibiotic should be used is after the patient has been given a chance to fight the invading germ and been unable to do so successfully – which should be apparent in an obvious deterioration in the patient's condition. Powerful drugs should only be used when absolutely essential, that is, very rarely. Otherwise the drug will kill other germs that naturally inhabit the throat, skin and bowel, and this can only harm patients, for anything that interferes with normal processes cannot be right. I have also collected evidence that antibiotics can retard the natural healing of the body tissues. This would not matter if the antibiotic was being used to cure pneumonia or other serious illness, because the cure takes only a few days or so, and once the patient is better his or her tissues will soon recover.

The first time I noted this bad side-effect was when a patient of mine had an operation for gall-stones. This was in the era when surgeons thought they could abolish the risk of septic complications after major surgery. He was given penicillin before and for some days following the operation. Surprisingly, his abdominal wound did not heal as quickly as is usual and, in fact, burst open seven days after the operation when some of the stitches were removed. There was no sepsis, the tissues looked normal and were restitched. Eventually all was well.

Although in principle I was opposed to the use of antibiotics unless the need for them was clinically demonstrated, I did not at that time associate antibiotics with slow healing. However, as time went by, the evidence accumulated, though I could never muster enough to support my suspicion. Some time later I had a patient with arthritis of the hip. She was a horsewoman with a very large riding school. During one of our many chats she mentioned the fact that many of her horses were subject to cuts and bruises around the legs. During the pre-antibiotics era, the horses would lick their wounds; sometimes the veterinary surgeon advised some kind of dressing and they recovered very quickly and with no fuss. Even those that needed stitches did well. When antibiotics came in, the vet started giving the horse jabs of penicillin as a matter of routine – to ensure, as he said, that the cuts did not go septic. The riding-school owner noticed after a while that all these injuries were taking much longer to heal than ever before. I suddenly realized that my suspicion about antibiotics had received independent and unsolicited support.

Antibiotics can also cause allergies in patients' bodies. This had been so frequently demonstrated that it is a universally accepted fact. Now we can begin to see a further possible cause in the increase of asthma since 1960, twelve years after the formation of the National Health Service ...

First, doctors are generally unaware that antibiotics are both unnecessary and possibly contributing to asthma. Worse, as has been shown, they continue to prescribe them to cure what they have mistakenly diagnosed as bronchitis, and must therefore find more drugs to suppress the asthma that they are causing. It is little wonder that the simple and effective ephedrine is hardly looked at now. Doctors are now blinded by a marvellous marketplace of new drugs, sprays and steroids – those arch maskers of symptoms and destroyers of natural resistance. It has been shown that skin affected by dermatitis and treated with cortisone products heals, but with a deterioration in its texture; the new skin is thinner and weaker and therefore more prone to breaking down again. Imagine what this same drug can do to delicate lung tissue after continual spraying.

Is all this true or false? I am sure my stance will be challenged by members of the profession, and you are entitled to ask. Let me first say that in all my years as a GP – at least thirty – I have only twice ever used an antibiotic on a child. The first time was when I was called out to a child with genuine pneumonia – not all parents rush to the doctor for nothing, as they are so often accused. The second was for acute mastoiditis. Both patients recovered in the course of time – not the next day.

Eight years ago I went to visit a 7-year-old boy who

was suffering from 'bronchitis'. The condition had been bad for over two years, during which time he had been given several long courses of antibiotics. He was hardly ever at school and was under the care of his doctor and a hospital. The child's state was so bad that his father had been considering giving up his job and going back to Ireland; there was no prospect of work, but he hoped that the green fields and pure air would help his only son to recover. When I examined the boy I had no doubt that he had asthma and not bronchitis, and that the child's ill-health was caused by antibiotics. I stopped all treatment and gave him a little ephedrine. Within two days he was much better, and the week after he was back at school. At sixteen he took several O levels and passed all of them. He has never needed a doctor from that day on. Although he came down with a bad bout of influenza at age sixteen, he recovered from it without the help of a doctor.

When you consider all this evidence together two lines of argument begin to emerge: prior to antibiotics the real problem was the psychological aspect of asthma; this has now been supplanted by the artificially created, drug-induced asthma. Until this is realized any form of psychological approach will not only fail to cure but may in fact aggravate the symptoms by making either the child or the parents, or both, the scapegoats for bad medical treatment.

I watched a television programme in the United States quite recently that dealt with the whole problem of treating asthma. The approach was based on the fact that asthma was an accepted physical disease which only the knowledge and wisdom of medical science could control. In this way the patients and their families were made totally dependent on doctors. Within this familiar context the doctors did some very sensible things. They encouraged and trained the children in groups not to succumb to their disability, by swimming and taking on other sports and activities. They showed that asthmatic children did not have to sit about doing nothing and getting more miserable. Meanwhile, the usual medical investigations and treatment were carried out. In these ways the children now knew what their physical capabilities were and how dependent on drug treatment they must be.

Many of the children were given freedom to air their views. It was quite remarkable to hear how much they understood about the problem of asthma, how grateful they were for the treatment and how trustingly they believed their medical advisers. However, two recurring themes were voiced by the children. The first was the fear of death, which they experienced in their asthmatic attacks. Nobody seems to have told them that asthmatic attacks such as they had never killed anyone. The second was their resentment at being abnormal.

This feeling abounded partly through the use of such drugs as cortisone, which retard physical growth, and partly because they were treated in special groups. As I watched those lovely articulate children trapped in a mental and medicinal fortress, I cried unashamedly for them. I wept also for their parents who not only had to share the misery of a disabled child, but so many of them also had to make crippling financial sacrifices. In these circumstances it would be very hard to persuade the patients that a whole new way of looking at their treatment was needed – unless it was given by those same doctors who had 'helped' them so far.

If I am right, that many of these children need never have reached this stage of asthma, and that many of them could still be rescued, then we are witnessing another example of Ivan Illich's idea that medicalization can cause ill-health. With regard to Illich: I am pleased to say that the very high opinion of his intellectual ability I expressed so many years ago has been confirmed quite recently by his appointment to the Advisory Committee to HRH the Prince of Wales.

I expect you will have noticed that I have not yet referred to air pollution as a possible cause of asthma. This is because it is dealt with in the next chapter by Dr D.L.J. Freed. You will find that he now has doubts about its importance. I have never been persuaded that air pollution is a real cause and that is why my mind remained open to other possibilities. Dr Jane Austin, writing in *The Archives of Diseases in Childhood*, found that asthma and wheeze are just as prevalent in the Scottish Highlands as in urban areas, and even more so in the Isle of Skye. You can't get much further away from smog than that!

In any event, the specific cause was not very important because all my patients recovered by developing their own immunity. It was the sudden increase in the number of cases, the severity of the disease and the mounting death rate that confirmed my suspicion: the misuse of antibiotics is the prime suspect in the sickening tragedy of asthma and its treatment today.

Hay Fever

Another allergic disease closely related to asthma is hay fever, whose main symptoms include irritation and watering of the eyes, frequent bouts of sneezing and coughing. Like any other disease, the symptoms vary from quite mild to very severe. It occurs in the springtime and is caused sometimes by moulds, but most commonly by pollen from flowers, trees and shrubs, which is carried by the wind, and which soon makes its presence felt in susceptible people. Rain makes the pollen weigh more so that it tends to fall to the ground more readily – thus on wet windless days the pollen count in the atmosphere will be at its lowest, and vice versa on dry windy days. This fact accounts for the variation of symptoms in individual sufferers on different days.

The main difference between the two conditions is that the reaction of the body to hay fever is confined to the eyes, nose, throat and larynx (voice box) known as the upper respiratory mechanism. By contrast asthma affects the bronchi and lungs, the lower respiratory mechanism. These facts may one day provide a clue for further investigation.

The first step in all cases of hay fever should be to avoid, as far as possible, the countryside and gardens. Beyond that, wearing suitable sunglasses to protect the eyes from direct contact with pollen, and taking a suitable antihistamine, often allows many of the milder cases to develop their own immunity within two or three years. In cases where the symptoms are more severe, a vaccine can be made from the offending pollens and moulds after testing the patient. This works in exactly the same way as any other vaccine: by starting the patient with very small doses and gradually increasing them, the body is educated gradually to develop its own immunity; by the time the air is thick with pollen in spring, the body can cope effectively and no symptoms develop. Though completely scientific, this method is time-consuming, and will not be fully effective unless completed before the hay fever season.

Some patients, therefore, may need to wait for some months.

Nowadays we have a vast array of atomizers, some containing steroids, which when sprayed into the nose and throat, will abolish the symptoms immediately. What more could a patient ask – instant relief! No more watering eyes, sneezing or coughing. Why suffer, take pills and undergo a boring course of vaccine during the winter? Unless some explanation is given to the patients they will never understand why this method is wrong. Well, the same reasoning applied earlier to asthma pertains here – the principle of allowing and helping the body to develop its own immunity without interfering with it. The local effect of these sprays on the mucous membrane, or lining, of the nose is damaging in that the tissues contract to such a degree that when the effect of the drug has worn off, a 'rebound' effect takes over – the mucous membrane becomes much more swollen and this in turn necessitates a further dose of spraying. A vicious circle of bad treatment is thus established that can be broken only by the disappearance of the pollen. An ear, nose and throat surgeon for whom I have always had the highest regard warned me many years ago of the inadvisability of using any form of local drugging of the nasal membrane; he saw it as a pernicious habit fraught with many complications. How right he was then and how much more so now that the ever-dangerous drug cortisone is so often used in the spray. It has been recently reported that in some patients treated in this way hay fever symptoms have persisted into November! This is surely prima-facie evidence that present-day treatment so reduces the patient's resistance that the illness is prolonged way beyond the period in which it would have subsided without treatment.

This is yet another example of accepted medical practice turning an illness into a disease. The extent of the damage done will come to light only in the passage of years, but it is doubtful that the cause will ever be recognized or acknowledged. The fault must forever lie in the patient; medical science is inviolable!

Just as asthma cases have increased in number so have those of hay fever. There are no figures available for Great Britain, but the United States reports 14.6 million hay fever cases, which is about 80 per cent higher than the asthma figures. The former Soviet Union stated categorically that they have a tremendous increase, so there is no reason to suppose that our figures would not show similar increases.

The answer to the problem must be the same: stop all this ill-advised and excessive treatment and return to a more sane scientific approach. Only when this has been tried and failed could one justify using sprays. Even under these circumstances the patient should be given full information about its disadvantages, so that they will use it as sparingly as possible or even opt to battle out the six weeks of what is only in many cases a relatively minor discomfort. A natural cure should never be ruled out.

3 Asthma: An Overview

In the previous chapter I propounded my views on the asthma problem. In order to give you a wider perspective of the current thinking on the condition, there will now follow extracts, almost verbatim, from a paper written by Dr David L.J. Freed, a former lecturer in immunology at Manchester University and lately an allergist in private practice.

I chose this paper because I have known Dr Freed for at least fifteen years. Three years ago he was my joint author on a book entitled *Understanding Arthritis*. We also shared a keen interest in asthma. He is now in his forties and I am in my late eighties, so we represent views from very different points on the age spectrum.

The two specific references to me were not in the original script but he has agreed to these minor amendments in order to emphasize our unanimity of purpose.

Although he is critical of the orthodox approach to the problem he does set it out very clearly and fairly. (Some of the passages may be rather technical but most are fairly intelligible to the layperson.)

'At this time when mortality rates from other chronic diseases are on the decline, clinical observations in recent years have demonstrated an increase in the mortality from asthma in several countries.'

Professor U. Serafini, Rome, 1992[1]

Until the 1950s asthma was not thought to be a life-threatening condition. Thus Osler, writing 100 years ago: 'Death during the attack is unknown'; the *Oxford Medicine* in 1920: 'Prognosis is excellent. The sensitive type probably never dies in an attack and the non-sensitive type rarely dies in an attack'; Coke, 1923: 'The prognosis with regard to longevity is notoriously good'; and Conybeare's textbook in 1929; 'It is doubtful whether death has ever been caused by uncomplicated asthma' (i.e. asthma without emphysema).[2–5]

What on earth is going on here? Here we are in 1992, in the grip of a worldwide epidemic of asthma deaths, and only a few years ago our clinical ancestors were calmly saying that it never happened. Were they all blind? It seems hardly likely, since death from asthma suffocation is a peculiarly horrifying spectacle, and the medical giants of the past were so impressed by the curious benignity of asthma that they all mentioned it.

Well, whatever, there is no doubt that within the last three decades we have witnessed a striking increase in asthma deaths, accompanied by a high rise in asthma cases and asthma hospitalisation.[1,6–16] The phenomenon troubles every doctor who sees asthma, and attempted explanations have been many. The International Consensus Report on the Diagnosis and Management of Asthma, issued recently by the National Institutes of

Health,[17] reflects the views of most conventional chest physicians in laying the blame squarely on 'underdiagnosis and inappropriate treatment' (shorthand for not enough steroids). But this is hardly an adequate explanation for the strange harmlessness of the same condition a couple of generations ago, when diagnosis and treatment were primitive and steroids were not used at all.

If we accept that for some reason asthma is now a potentially fatal condition, even though it was not so in the recent past, then the physicians' call for earlier hospitalisation and more aggressive steroid treatment does appear reasonable. But we still have a duty to ask why asthma cases have increased so dramatically and become more fatal. There are two disturbing factors which may provide answers: (i) air pollution has vastly increased over the last few decades; (ii) the drugs which are used to control asthma may actually be making the condition worse long term.

The views that I am about to expound are my own, but the data on which they are based are public property and verifiable by anyone with access to a public library who can check citations at the end of this essay. Ten years ago I was shouted off the rostrum by a group of chest physicians to whom I had predicted that we would soon be experiencing a further rise in asthma deaths. The reasons for the physicians' hostility may become apparent as we proceed. My grim prediction can now be seen, in 1992, to be coming true, although I cannot take much pleasure in that vindication.

Recognized Risks

There is no doubt that air pollution, both natural and man-made, is a major contributor to illness and death from asthma.[18] The classic artificial pollutant was the great 1952 winter fog which killed 4,000 Londoners.[18] Among 'natural' pollutants are included the dust of soya beans, which causes a mini-epidemic at the port of Cartagena, Spain, on unloading days.[19] Probably the most famous natural pollutant, the house-dust mite (*Dermatophagoides pteronyssinus*) and its minute faecal particles, is much more prevalent in modern homes because of greater warmth, insulation and fitted carpets.[20] Energy-saving construction of houses has much to answer for; a house that keeps in heat also tends to keep in pollutants. Lastly, one must not forget that one can be allergic to viruses, as well as being infected by them, and infection by one of the common respiratory viruses is a proven asthma trigger in susceptible persons;[21] no one, however, has suggested that viruses are commoner now than in generations past.

There is, however, another pollutant proposed persuasively by Dr William W. Fox: antibiotics commonly prescribed for babies and children who are thought by GPs to suffer from possible serious infection. He argues his own case and I believe he may be right.

As regards anti-asthma drugs, most concern has focused on the group of drugs called beta-agonists, starting with isoprenaline in the 1960s and continuing with the new generation of 'safe', non-cardiotoxic analogues such as Ventolin and

Serovent.[22–27] Regular use of these drugs gives rise to a substantial rebound phenomenon when they are withdrawn,[28] and increases the so-called 'non-specific' reactivity of asthmatic airways, e.g. reactions to methacholine or histamine.[22] Tachyphylaxis occurs, at least in vitro – that is, larger and larger doses are required to obtain the same degree of bronchodilatation.[22] Furthermore, these drugs disrupt magnesium metabolism which in turn aggravates smooth-muscle lability.[29] In practice, at least one chest expert now tries to wean his patients off long-term beta-agonists, explaining that they 'keep your asthma active'.[30] Continuous beta-agonist bronchodilatation causes long-term deterioration of lung function.[31] Intermittent (on-demand) treatment is less dangerous in this respect[31] and I have found that even nebulizer-dependent patients can often tolerate a 'sabbatical' break from treatment one day a week, with what I hope will be an improved long-term prognosis.

After the upsurge in asthma deaths in the mid 1960s, which included well-publicized cases such as that of Brian Jones, the Rolling Stone, there was a general perception among the public that asthma inhalants were dangerous; drug consumption fell and mortality fell. By the mid 1970s physicians had regained their confidence with the new generation of 'safe' bronchodilators and prescription rates started rising again, to be followed shortly by death rates.[7] This fall and subsequent rise in mortality rates does rather argue against the 'increased pollution' theory, since air pollution (at least the carboniferous variety) was rising pretty smoothly throughout those years.[32]

Asthma is common. Eleven per cent of all children have wheezy episodes, which if managed by Dr Fox's method will often resolve quite quickly or which (if left alone) normally resolve by the age of 10.[33] The worry is that by calling these wheezy episodes 'asthma' and thus triggering the doctor's prescribing reflex (*'furor therapeuticus'*), we might convert a benign transient wheeze into a chronic condition that needs ever-increasing drug intake to keep it under control. To quote one recent Canadian view, 'We should hesitate before recommending regular use of beta-agonists',[27] or to borrow the even more provocative words of one group of New Zealand asthmatologists in 1992: 'Is the cure the cause?'[11]

Pathology

Many autopsies have been carried out on patients who have died of asthma. Two types of picture emerge. The most common is widespread plugging of the bronchi and bronchioles with thick mucus, often so thick and hard it cannot be sucked up with a pipette but has to be cut with a knife. The mucus plug forms a perfect cast of the inner shape of the air tube and is obviously the main cause of suffocation.[1] Embedded in the mucus are numerous inflammatory cells (neutrophils and eosinophils), together with clumps or even sheets of epithelial cells (the cells which normally line the inner surface). These patients have usually died in hospital after several days or weeks of increasingly aggressive treatment.[34] On the other hand there are those who die unexpectedly, in their homes or at work, and in these cases the airways are often empty on post-mortem, having relaxed after death from the tight and sudden bronchoconstriction that was the presumed cause of death.[34]

What is Going on in Asthma?

The wheezing of asthma is caused by narrowing of the bronchi and bronchioles. This is caused by inflammation.[35] Inflammation is the body's defence and repair mechanism for coping with 'insults' from the environment such as germs, harmful chemicals, extremes of heat and cold, radiation and physical traumata. Inflammation at mucous surfaces in the body shares the characteristics of inflammation in solid organs (dilatation of blood vessels, migration of inflammatory cells from blood to interstitial fluid) and also has two characteristics of its own: increased mucous secretion (containing some of the said inflammatory cells) and shedding (desquamation) of sheets of epithelium.[35] Clearly, these two features serve to trap particles and chemicals and carry them away from the sensitive membrane underneath, rather like the continuous shedding of the surface cells that occurs normally in the skin and gut.

Allergy, in immunologists' terminology, is an immunological process that leads to inflammation. That is to say, by this definition, allergy is one of the body's natural defence mechanisms. And therefore according to this line of thought (which is fully in accordance with conventional biological thinking, albeit rarely followed to its logical conclusion by clinicians) asthma itself must be protective in some way, against some insult. Mother nature did not put smooth muscle into our bronchi just in order to make mischief, and this is why I have preached for the last decade the need for clear terminology;[36] 'allergy' means different things to different people, but our attitude to symptoms that reflect a bodily defence mechanism may well be different from our attitude to symptoms brought about by straightforward poisoning.

When the highways department decides to repair a stretch of motorway, it closes some of the carriageways and considerable congestion results while the repairs get done. In extreme cases the engineers may close the entire width of the motorway for a while and traffic simply has to stop or use another route. The bronchi may be looked upon in the same light. For repairs to be carried out on the air tubes, it may have to be narrowed or completely stopped for a while. Total airflow is of course restricted, although the chest has considerable spare capacity and gas exchange in the lungs is not seriously embarrassed until terminal stages. Moreover, when the airways are narrowed another effect occurs, mostly unnoticed as all the attention is focused on the sensation of breathlessness and the effort required to breathe. Although the amount of air passing through that stretch of bronchus may be reduced, its velocity and turbulence are increased,[37] giving rise to a 'scouring' action that would encourage the mucus (and any particles or chemicals trapped therein) to become detached from the inner wall of the bronchus and be forced upwards towards the throat. This effect would be seriously compromised by any drug which permitted the secretion of mucus but prevented it from being carried away (by preventing, in this view, the bronchoconstriction that sets up the scouring). Beta-agonists certainly would be expected to do this, and at first sight it would seem that we must support the belief of most chest physicians that glucocorticoids ('steroids') should be used more aggressively, since steroids suppress inflammation. But there are four main snags to the use of steroids: (i) steroids, even the inhaled variety, are just too dangerous;[38] (ii) they don't always work,[39] as for instance when the inflammation is caused not by an immune reaction but by direct toxicity (see below); and (iii) not all mucous secretion is caused by inflammation. It can also be stimulated by certain plant toxins called lectins (the mucotractive effect)[40] and there are lectins a-plenty in pollen grains and presumably in other allergenic particles.[41] Steroids would not be expected to stop mucous secretion by that mechanism; they would merely prevent the mucus from being coughed up. The mucus would stay in the airway, getting dryer and stickier.

And even (iv) if we could find the perfect drug, that entirely suppresses not only inflammation (both immune and toxic types) but also mucus secretion (both inflammatory and mucotractive types), so that mucous plugging and asthma fatalities were abolished (I do just wonder whether cromoglycate might not fall into this category, for those cases in which it works,[42]) it would still in theory leave the body open to pollen and mite toxins (not necessarily allergens), which would probably exert effects on distant, non-pulmonary sites and might even be worse.

Allergens and Toxins
All these considerations lead me to conclude that asthma, like other forms of inflammation, is actually a natural self-cleaning and repair mechanism for the bronchi. But what exactly is the chest protecting itself against? Germs, noxious gases and airborne plant toxins are obviously 'bad things' that should be removed as far as possible from the body, but what about allergens such as pollen grains, mould spores, foods and *Dermatophagoides* droppings?

My experiments with pollen grains and house-dust mites showed a startling degree of toxicity.[43] A single pollen grain can destroy about 100 red blood cells by its soluble, low molecular weight toxins (probably plant amino acids). *Dermatophagoides* are just as bad. Pollen toxins, extracted and purified from all antigens (and thus incapable of causing an immune response) caused tissue damage and inflammation when injected into healthy skin, and this inflammation was not suppressed by steroids.[43] Plant toxins are frequently small molecules, like the pollen toxins that I described. They are too small to be noticed by the immunological system, although they can still poison the tissues. They sneak in, as it were, under the guard of the immune system. Fortunately for us, nature usually packages them in large-ish particles (like pollen grains and mould spores), and these also contain large molecules which the body does recognize. While the particles are in contact with the mucous membrane they cause considerable damage just by being there,[44,45] stripping away surface cells, exposing nerve endings and thus contributing to the non-specific irritability that is the hallmark of asthmatic airways.[35] But eventually the immune inflammation drives the whole particle and its soluble products out of the body (though at the cost of causing symptoms). We must therefore be very cautious about using drugs that prevent this natural defence mechanism.

Foods, amazingly, can also be poisonous (albeit only slowly); most if not all of the vegetable kingdom possesses intrinsic natural poisons, some of them very toxic indeed (like the microdose of ricin on the tip of the poisoned umbrella that killed Gyorgi Markov – ricin is extracted from castor-oil seeds.[46]) The only essential difference between, say, tomatoes on the one hand and deadly nightshade on the other is the dose of poison in them; tomatoes contains small amounts and belladonna has rather more.[46] The field of food toxicology has been well known to farmers and vets for a century or more, but is only now dimly reaching the consciousness of medics.

At first sight it is difficult to believe a role for foods in asthma. Airborne particles and chemicals are one thing, they hit the lung directly, but how can foods be involved? The connection is more intimate than one would think. Because of their innate toxicity, foods are 'filtered' three times before they enter the bloodstream. Firstly in the intestines, which suffers a huge loss of epithelial cells daily in the process but should, in health, succeed in digesting all proteins and carbohydrates to a state of harmlessness. Next to the liver, where the cytochrome P450 system of enzymes detoxifies those poisons (drugs, chemicals, other xenobiotics) that have evaded digestion in the gut. And lastly, via the portal vein and the right side of the heart, to the lungs, where any residual poisons and particles should be ingested by phagocytic cells and where, if an extra excretion step is required, those cells can be passed into the air spaces of the lung for expulsion via 'the mucous escalator'. It should be remembered that *fats* and fat-soluble poisons bypass the first two filters (gut and liver) altogether as they are absorbed direct into the lymph and thus pass straight to the lungs. Their intimate relationship with lymphocytes during that journey will make another story another time. The lung therefore is deeply concerned in the final elimination of dietary poisons, as befits one of the major interfaces between body and environment and the same considerations apply to foods as to inhaled poisons.

It is worth considering in parentheses the action of antibiotics. These are the only drugs in the pharmacopoeia that act not on the body but on the invading particles. They are the outstanding success story of the 20th century, a shining example of how the study of aetiology (causes) can reap far greater rewards than the study of pathogenesis (mechanisms). Modern clinical immunologists, unlike their predecessors of the first part of the century, are unique in turning their attention to suppressing the patient's immunology rather than utilizing it in his defence.

The Unwelcome Conclusion

It is we the doctors who have turned asthma into a killer.

Any drug, be it a beta-agonist or any other class, that effectively reverses constriction and inflammation of the airways, must render the patient more susceptible to the direct toxic effects of the particles and chemicals that that inflammation was trying to remove and is therefore likely to increase mortality. This effect will be in direct proportion to the drug's effectiveness at relieving symptoms. The physicians' approach (prescribing physic) – if effective – must inevitably cause deaths, and the apparent harmlessness of asthma up to the recent past is because the medicines used in those days were ineffective. (Give any doctor powerful drugs and he starts killing patients.)

It may be that in acute emergency situations, beta-agonists and other drugs are life-saving. But in the long term we simply have no evidence other than the rising epidemic of asthma deaths, because no long-term trials have ever been done, or will ever be done, in which treated asthmatics are compared to untreated asthmatics. This is because most doctors cannot ethically bring themselves to randomize any asthmatic into a placebo or non-intervention group. There are simply no untreated asthmatics. To put it starkly, the long-term management of asthma is one huge uncontrolled experiment, the results of which we are witnessing today but which we cannot agree about because it is uncontrolled.

The hostility of my physician audience 10 years

ago is based on the fact that although they were doing their conscientious best, their patients were dying in greater and greater numbers, and their policies were (and still are) based not on science but on inarticulate hypothesis, pious hope and persuasive advertising by the drug companies. (The April 1992 issue of the *Journal of Allergy and Clinical Immunology*, which is read by all American and most British allergists, contained, I noticed, 112 pages of scientific text, 9 pages of public announcements and 50 pages of brightly coloured drug ads. Hmmm.) In retrospect I could not have expected the physicians to take kindly to a cocky youngster from a new scientific discipline breezing in and telling them that they had been doing it wrong all along.

So What Do We Do Instead?
1) You could try to identify the offending substances and try to avoid them. In practical terms this could begin before birth, with pregnant mothers avoiding the commonest food allergens, continuing avoidance during lactation and at the same time reducing the Dermatophagoides levels in the home by well-established house-cleansing methods.[48,49] Although laborious this regimen does prevent much allergy in genetically susceptible babies.[49] In this context we should pause for a moment to consider the role of *milk* in asthma, particularly pasteurised, homogenized, bovine 'doorstep' milk as consumed universally in the Anglo-Saxon countries (UK, Australia, New Zealand, USA and Canada). These are precisely the countries with the highest prevalence of asthma.[7]

Milk is the commonest food to cause food allergy, presumably because its consumption is so widespread and begins so early in life. Milk also has a non-specific sensitizing effect, so that even if you are not actually allergic to milk, it will make you more sensitive to other allergens such as Dermatophagoides, for example, if you are allergic to that.[50,51] Morrow Brown has reported a case of a dust-allergic child with no evidence of milk sensitivity who nevertheless got better when milk was avoided,[52] and in an unpublished series of 10 asthmatic children studied at the Manchester Royal Infirmary I found the same phenomenon; 5 out of the 10 were 'cured' by the simple expedient of adopting a dairy-free diet, even though none of the 10 had any evidence of allergy to milk itself. Since that experience I have adopted the rule of putting all asthmatics on a dairy-free regimen first of all (there is plenty of calcium in fish, eggs etc.). Only if that regimen is insufficient do I go on to other interventions.

Curiously, the Japanese (who consume hardly any milk because of their genetic inability to digest lactose after infancy) have an asthma prevalence of one twentieth of ours,[7] although in fairness it should be added that they have far less dust in their homes.[53]

(2) You could try to enlist the aid of the patient's immune system instead of suppressing it, by some kind of immunization. The body has other defence systems apart from inflammation, for example the secretory IgA antibody system, which protects without inflammation. Although it is not clear how

the various types of desensitization work, they all involve the administration of antigen in some form and could well be having some effect of this kind. The evidence for this is strong in the case of conventional hyposensitization, which evokes 'blocking antibodies' among other things; I am not aware that the newer forms of desensitization (neutralization and EPD) have been adequately studied in this regard. Although these methods are far safer than conventional hyposensitization in the short term, we still lack the very long term follow-up studies that are needed to see if they are associated with mortality. Nevertheless, experience so far is comforting.

Neutralization, for example, is in routine use by over 3,000 doctors in North America and has so far not been associated with a single mortality,[54] unlike conventional hyposensitization and drugs which emphatically have.

(3) You can in the meantime use Dr Fox's treatment to produce early and satisfying results. If he is right then his meticulous attention to all the detail of the history of asthma will be vindicated. This could mean that much expensive scientific research and treatment can be discontinued.

What I hope you will have gleaned from this contribution are:

1. That there are toxins, allergens or possibly viruses that could be responsible for some cases of asthma. Although this possibility was fully considered in the early part of the 1900s, no research since has succeeded

in identifying a single cause for the disease. It is therefore likely that we are chasing a red herring whilst there are many small sprats which may have a minor but important role in different cases. This is true in probably a third of the cases – those who recovered without treatment in the old days and in spite of treatment in modern times, because the natural defence mechanisms of the patient had succeeded.

My chief concern, however, is to explain the new factor that accounts for the enormous increase in asthmatic cases and the condition's severity. Let us return to Dr Freed's description of the tragic state of the bronchi and lungs in patients who have died. As I have indicated under 'Teething' and 'Infection' many children are given antibiotics when they show evidence of what the GP thinks is infection such as a high temperature, inflammation of the middle ear and wheezing or coughing which he all too easily thinks is bronchitis. There is a consensus amongst consultants that almost half the number of GPs have difficulty in distinguishing bronchitis and asthma.

It is at this point that those patients who are allergic to the antibiotic will become worse because the antibiotic will generate the body's normal reaction which is the wheezing syndrome.

This situation now compels the doctors to try to improve the patient's condition. This sometimes entails removal to hospital and oxygen tents and the increased use of steroids and beta-agonists. Thus a vicious circle is established in which, in extreme cases, the body loses its power to resist and the bronchi become choked. In a few cases death ensues.

2. Most drugs in daily use have some side-effects that

can be very serious. Any form of steroid falls within that category, in my view. Beta-agonists in particular are now suspected actually to trigger off new attacks. Read this extract from a report in *The Times* of 1 October 1993:

A drug widely prescribed for asthma increases sensitivity to allergens such as pollens and cat fur, scientists have found.

The drug salbutamol, also prescribed to Britain's three million asthma sufferers under the trade name Ventolin, doubles the sensitivity to allergens when taken regularly and could pose a serious risk to patients with severe asthma according to a study in the *Lancet*.

More than 2,000 patients die from asthma each year and the number diagnosed with the condition is increasing. Fears have grown in recent years that inappropriate use of asthma drugs might have contributed to the rise in the death rate. In the *Lancet* study, patients taking salbutamol regularly for two weeks became more sensitive to allergens. The protective effect of the drug also decreased over the period.

The study, by researchers in Nottingham and Canada, will add to fears about the regular use of the beta-2 agonist class of drugs, such as salbutamol. Four years ago a study in New Zealand showed that regular use of fenoterol, another beta-2 agonist, increased the risk of death.

The researchers say that salbutamol and similar drugs should be used only occasionally to ward off an attack of wheezing. Patients whose asthma is more severe and who need regular treatment to prevent attacks should use an inhaled steroid drug, they say.

Melinda Letts, director of the National Asthma Campaign, said that many patients were failing to take a steroid prescribed with salbutamol. 'Anyone who is using a relieving drug such as salbutamol more than once a day should be using a steroid preventer medicine as well.'

Let me now give you a thumbnail sketch of the steroid's history.

In 1949 reporters from the world's press gathered for a conference on Fifth Avenue, New York, where leading American rheumatologists announced that they had discovered a cure for rheumatoid arthritis. Patients crippled by the disease were able to get out of their wheelchairs and run, never mind walk, across the room. Within a year the news gradually leaked out that the same patients were now in much worse a condition than they had ever been before the cure. An overdose of the drug was deemed the main reason. The treatment was more or less abandoned, but over the years variations of the steroid have been developed and cautiously used to alleviate rheumatoid arthritis. While relatively small doses gave some relief to patients, even this was short-lived. In fact the passage of time showed that in spite of short-term relief the disease progressed at a more rapid rate than it did in untreated patients.

Steroids are still used by rheumatologists in order to make patients 'more comfortable' during difficult periods, and when they go into a natural remission the dose can be reduced or stopped. I have categorically refused to use these drugs, because the relief offered to patients only flatters to deceive, while the deterioration of bodily tissues and defence mechanisms marches on relentlessly. In the case of rheumatoid arthritis, steroids do not pose any immediate threat to life. But in giving relief the drug suppresses the body's inflammatory reaction – a natural defence mechanism of the body and the real cause of the pain – so allowing the disease to develop unhindered and, in the process giving rise to further damage to the joints.

In the parallel treatment of asthma, the same immediate relief is produced by the steroid, but bronchial and lung tissue deteriorates at a more rapid rate, so that sooner or later, the patient cannot cope with the breathing necessary to maintain life, so death becomes inevitable. A key difference, however, is between the deterioration in a joint which is not vital to life and that of the bronchi and lungs which are.

What conclusions can we reasonably draw from the material contained in these chapters?

1. The incidence of asthma has increased from a maximum of 100,000 cases per anum before the 1960s to about 3 million in the 1990s.
2. Deaths from asthma have steadily risen from about 1,000 in the 1970s to well over 2,000 in the 1990s.
3. There were no known deaths from asthma before the 1960s, but they began to appear in the 1960s.
4. Antibiotics became freely available after 1948, the year the National Health Service was established.
5. Antibiotics were given to babies when a severe infection was suspected by the doctor.
6. General practitioners were not, and still probably are not, aware of the harmless nature of the teething syndrome.
7. There is no evidence of any significant drop in the death rate of babies up to three years old between

the 1940s and the 1960s that could not be attributed to the rising standards of food and housing.

8. This suggests that the widespread use of antibiotics did not save a significant number of lives.

9. Pollutants are often proposed as a cause of asthma, but they have been with us since the Industrial Revolution. The widespread smog of the industrial North and Midlands caused bronchitis in older people, but asthma remained rare.

10. Exhaust fumes and man-made pollutants in the environment may all be partly responsible but with reasonable care most of the problems they cause can be minimized by asthma sufferers.

11. Toxins and allergens in food and viruses may play a role, but so must they have done when asthma was rare and deaths unknown. This is proof enough of what natural resistance can achieve without medical treatment.

12. Whatever arguments are made in favour of present-day treatment and its results, their value must be weighed against the evidence and experience of my lifelong career: not a single case of asthma in the first three years of life that came under my care failed to recover completely in a very short time.

With the few children who came my way when they were established asthmatics between the ages of four and twelve I stopped antibiotics, and reduced other treatment gradually so as to avoid rebound and addictions problems – indeed they all recovered and lived normal lives soon after I took charge.

You the readers are now informed of my views and

treatment. You can now disprove or attest to the reliability of what I have written by answering the following questionnaire:

Name: **Age:** **Sex:**

Address:

1. At what age were you diagnosed as asthmatic?

2. At what age were you first given antibiotics?

3. What reason did the doctor give for prescribing it?

4. How many times were you given antibiotics, over what period of time, and for what reasons?

5. Were you worried about the asthma and ever frightened about the possibility of dying from the disease?

6. Were you ever told that asthma was not a fatal disease and that complete recovery was possible?

7. Have you ever sought alternative medicine? If so, what, why and with what results?

8. In your opinion, do you think what I have described in this book resembles your experience or not? If you do not agree, please state your reason.

Robert Hale, the publishers, will forward to me all your replies, which will be analysed and assessed. Please enclose a stamped, addressed envelope, so that we can notify you of the results when they become available.

You will appreciate that the custodians of medical ethics would soon be branding me as irresponsible if I told you what course of treatment to adopt. In some of you asthma will be so far advanced that a sudden cessation of your current treatment could be life-threatening. I cannot advise you what to do without your own doctor's agreement.

There must surely be some general practitioners who are unhappy with present-day treatment – let's hope yours is one who might listen with an open mind. This is perhaps the only way for these new concepts to gain support. As I stated earlier, efforts by individual writers cannot hope for a lasting effect. They must be backed up by an organization that speaks out the truth, loud and clear, until the medical establishment takes positive steps to investigate. The media now has a real opportunity to serve the public in a tangible and praiseworthy way.

But what about the misery and suffering and deaths which can be largely eliminated? Despite the number of charities pleading for help with natural and man-made disasters all over the world, a little attention to the asthma disaster would not be out of place. Indeed the irony is that the problem does not really need money, for a change of treatment philosophy will save considerable amounts! The Treasury ought to be interested in reducing the cost of treating asthma – £1.75 billion per year and rising. What a figure. I urge you to persuade the media to take an active interest in this devastating problem. Remember what I said in the preface: 'The terrible tragedy is that they [doctors] do not consciously exploit the public, nor are they criminals; they genuinely believe they are efficient and honest. This kind of thinking ... will change only as the result of a mental revolution.'

This book has all the necessary ingredients: spark off the revolution with your hearts and minds.

The final chapter will demonstrate what I have had to contend with since my book *Arthritis: Is Your Suffering Really Necessary?* was published in 1981. Success for those ideas may well be on the way. Don't allow success for this book to take so long.

4   Resolution

You may wonder why this book has not been written before, and why the medical profession seem to be so ignorant about the problem. I have already referred to the difficulties I encountered in trying to get my work published, but I have selected a few highlights to give a clear insight into the opposition I faced.

You will remember that in the introduction I discussed the work of Dr David Horrobin, Professor Ian Kennedy and Ivan Illich and their criticisms of the medical profession. To these three I must now add Dr Donald Gould, a medical journalist who wrote a book entitled *The Medical Mafia*. There is no need to quote from it because the title is enough to convey his views, but it can still be purchased in paperback. Dr Vernon Coleman, originally a GP, is another author who has written numerous books on medical subjects over the last thirty years. One of them is *The Health Scare – Your Health in Crisis*. What he has to say about the medical profession is best quoted from an article of his in the *European Medical Journal*, of which he is the editor. Entitled 'Doctors Do More Harm Than Good', it is reproduced in full here.

Doctors save lives but they also kill people.

There is nothing new in that.

Doctors have always made mistakes and there have always been patients who have died as a result of medical ignorance or incompetence.

But we have now reached the point where, on balance, well meaning doctors in general practice and highly trained, well equipped specialists working in hospitals do more harm than good. Through a mixture of ignorance and incompetence doctors are killing more people than they are saving, and they are causing more illness and more discomfort than they are alleviating.

It is true, of course, that doctors save thousands of lives by prescribing life saving drugs like antibiotics, and by performing essential life saving surgery on accident victims.

But this good is far outweighed by the bad, and the epidemic of iatrogenic disease (disease caused by doctors) which has scarred medical practice for decades has been steadily getting worse. Today most of us would, most of the time, be better off without a medical profession.

Not long ago the former Director General of the World Health Orgnization startled the medical establishment by stating that 'the major and most expensive part of medical knowledge as applied today appears to be more for the satisfaction of the health professions than for the benefit of the consumers of health care'. The evidence certainly supports that apparently controversial view.

Just look at the facts.

In America there is one doctor for every 452 people and life expectancy for black males is 65.5 years. In Jamaica there is one doctor for every 7,033 people and life expectancy for men is 69.2 years. In North Korea there is one doctor for every 417 patients and life expectancy for males is 63 years. In South Korea there is one doctor for every 1,509 people and life expectancy is 64.9 years. Those figures hardly support the image of doctors as an effective healing profession.

Even more startling, perhaps, is the evidence of what happens when doctors go on strike and leave patients to cope without professional medical help. You might imagine that people would be dying like flies in autumn. Not a bit of it. When doctors in Israel went on strike for a month, admissions to hospital dropped by eighty-five per cent, with only the most urgent cases being admitted. But despite this fall the death rate in Israel dropped by fifty per cent – the largest drop since the previous doctors' strike twenty years earlier – to its lowest ever recorded level. Much the same thing has happened wherever doctors have gone on strike. In Bogota, Colombia, doctors went on strike for fifty-two days and there was a thirty-five per cent fall in the mortality rate. In Los Angeles a doctors' strike resulted in an eighteen per cent reduction in the death rate. During the strike there were sixty per cent fewer operations in seventeen major hospitals. After the strike was over the death rate went back up to normal.

Whatever statistics are consulted the conclusion has to be the same: doctors are a hazard rather than an asset to any community. In Britain the death rate of working men over fifty years of age was higher in the 1970s than it was in the 1930s. The British were never healthier than they were during the Second World War. Figures published by the United States Bureau of Census show that thirty-three per cent of the people born in 1907 could expect to live to the age of seventy-five whereas thirty-three per cent of the people born in 1977 could expect to live to the age of eighty. Remove the improvements produced by better living conditions, cleaner water supplies, and fewer deaths during or just after childbirth and it becomes clear that doctors, drug companies and hospitals cannot possibly have had any useful effect on life expectancy. Indeed, the figures show that there has been an increase in mortality rates among the middle aged and an increase in the incidence of disabling disorders such as diabetes and arthritis.

Could there be some other explanation for this dispiriting phenomenon? Hardly. When you look at the quality of medical care it becomes clear that it must be doctors who are responsible for the decline in health. The amount of ignorance among doctors is staggering.

Writing in the *Postgraduate Medical Journal* two pathologists reported that after carrying out 400 post mortem examinations they found that in more than half of the patients the wrong diagnosis had been made. The two pathologists reported that potentially treatable disease was missed in one in seven patients. They found that sixty-five out of one hundred and thirty-four cases of pneumonia had gone unrecognized while out of fifty-one patients who had suffered heart attacks doctors had failed to diagnose the problem in eighteen cases.

A study of GPs reported in a medical newspaper showed that a quarter of general practitioners do not know about the connection between smoking and heart disease while, amazingly, twenty per cent of GPs are unaware that cigarettes can cause lung cancer. From France comes evidence that in the final examinations for medical students in Paris one tenth of the candidates made no mention of tobacco when asked to list factors responsible for causing cancer. By contrast well over a third of the students mentioned the type of cancer produced in horses' mouths by the rubbing of the bit.

Dr Badal Pal, Senior Registrar in the Department of Rheumatology at Dryburn Hospital, Durham, questioned seventy general practitioners and found that half of them knew little about the ingredients of popular non steroidal anti-inflammatory drugs – probably the most commonly used drugs in medicine today, and taken regularly by millions of arthritis sufferers.

A survey conducted by the Royal College of General Practitioners showed that many experienced family doctors had inadequate knowledge about the diagnosis and treatment of common disorders. Questionnaires which were posted to 1,400 general practitioners included questions about common conditions such as anaemia, middle ear infection, glandular fever and jaundice but according to Dr William Acheson, Senior Lecturer in General Practice at Manchester University, many of the doctors who responded 'failed to mention answers that were important. Some gave unusual answers and some gave answers that were clearly wrong.' Only half the doctors in the survey mentioned the three most common symptoms in middle ear infection. More than half left out important questions to ask a patient with jaundice. Dr Donald Alastair Donald, Chairman of the Joint Committee for Postgraduate Training in General Practice, said that he was not surprised by the deficiencies revealed in the report. 'All knowledge dissipates at a steady rate unless it is topped up,' he said. 'The average general practitioner spends only four hours a year at postgraduate courses.'

The consequences of all this ignorance are appalling. Dr Gareth Beevers, a physician at the Dudley Road Hospital in Birmingham, England, and a lecturer in medicine at Birmingham University, estimates that around one in eight patients in hospital are there because of problems caused by drugs they have been given by their doctors. Dr Patrick Pietroni, Senior Lecturer in General Practice at St Mary's Hospital Medical School in London, thinks the figure is even higher, he reports that one in six patients in hospital are there because of some side effect of their medication. All the evidence shows that doctors simply do not know very much about the drugs they prescribe.

It has been known since 1961 that the benzodiazepine drugs are addictive. The problem was first described in 1973 – and predicted that benzodiazepine addiction would be a massive problem within a few years. In the mid 1980s it was estimated that there were three million benzo-diazepine addicts in Britain alone. And yet even today – in 1992 – there are still doctors who are handing out prescriptions for benzodiazepines who insist that these drugs are perfectly safe, are not addictive and can be taken – and stopped – without any worry.

But it is not only family doctors who need to be better trained. A report published in the *Journal of the Royal Society of Medicine* concluded that many hospital patients who suffer heart attacks die during the 'confused and disorganised charades' of attempts to save them because hospital doctors do not know how to give emergency resuscitation. According to the report, which surveyed fifty junior hospital doctors, only four doctors were able to perform effectively when asked to demonstrate their skills on a model.

Even more worrying was an editorial published in the *British Medical Journal* in October 1991 which stated that 'only one per cent of the articles in medical journals are scientifically sound' and that 'only about fifteen per cent of medical interventions are supported by solid scientific evidence'. In other words, the majority of treatments are completely untried and when a doctor writes out a prescription or sticks a knife into a patient neither he nor anyone else has much of an idea about what will happen next.

Not that this epidemic of incompetence is entirely professional. Much of the illness caused by doctors (and by nurses) is a consequence of a more basic type of ignorance.

For example, at least one in twenty of all hospital patients will pick up an infection in hospital – mostly urinary tract, chest or wound infections and mostly caused by doctors and nurses failing to wash their hands often enough. Since Ignaz

Philipp Semmelweiss first demonstrated (in the mid nineteenth century) that deaths in the delivery room were caused by dirty hands every child has been taught the importance of basic personal hygiene. Sadly, it seems that the message does not seem to have got through to the medical and nursing professions. A study of five British hospitals in 1984 showed that nurses washed their hands only once every three times after cleaning around a patient's catheter while three years later a study at a hospital in the North of England showed that hand-washing by staff was well below levels recommended by the United States Centres for Disease Control guidelines. Similar studies in America have found that two out of three anaesthetists failed to wash their hands before treating a new patient (even though anaesthetists frequently perform venepuncture surgery), while one in three surgeons did not wash their arms properly before an operation.

At least one third of all hospital infections are caused by dirty hands and the cost in simple financial terms is colossal (though not, of course, as horrendous or as unforgivable as the cost in human terms). In Britain hospital infections cost the National Health Service well over £100 million a year – and 950,000 lost bed days. It is hardly surprising that waiting lists for treatment are long. And it is hardly surprising that people who stay at home to be treated – or who go home quickly after a day case or short stay surgery – usually get better much quicker than people who need long term in-hospital treatment.

There are many reasons why doctors are

currently doing so much harm to their patients, but the most important is undoubtedly the fact that while doctors are now in possession of technologies and techniques which are powerful, the profession's relationship with patients is still based on the theory that in order to do good the average doctor must rely on fear and respect.

When doctors didn't have powerful drugs they relied heavily upon the mystique of being a 'doctor'. The mysticism and the witchcraft long associated with the practice of medicine was an important part of the healing process. Because he knew that the pills and potions he prescribed had very little intrinsic value a doctor had to convince his patients that he knew what he was doing and that he had faith that the remedies he was using would work. The doctor knew that if his patients believed that they were going to get better then many of them would – even if they were only given some primitive and entirely useless concoction. The power of the placebo is well documented – and even quite severe pains can be controlled with sugar pills if the doctor giving them out is convincing.

Giving the patient a prescription was an important ritual; it was offering the patient a part of the doctor to take with him, and the important thing was to get the patient to believe that it would do him some good. The old fashioned witch doctors were fearful. So were Victorian physicians and surgeons. Patients accepted what their doctors told them as though it was gospel.

But today doctors have powerful and potentially lethal drugs and treatments at their disposal, and the old fashioned mystique is dangerous. Modern drugs can save lives but they are so powerful that they can – and frequently do – also cause problems. Research has shown that approximately forty per cent of all patients who are prescribed drug treatment suffer severe or noticeable side effects.

Patients can be too easily tempted to ask for (or expect) drugs and doctors can far too easily trick themselves into thinking that a prescription is necessary.

When drugs were ineffective and harmless it didn't matter if doctors gave out drugs to every patient they saw. (Indeed, the apothecaries – the original general practitioners – had to give drugs to all their patients since they earned their living through dispensing and were not allowed to charge fees simply for providing advice.)

But today, although drugs are so powerful that they should be used cautiously and only when absolutely essential, old habits still persist and four out of five consultations in general practice end with the doctor handing over a prescription (although far fewer patients expect to get a prescription and most would almost certainly be happier if they left the surgery without one). The result is that we have become a nation of pill swallowers. At any one time six out of ten people will be taking a drug of some kind. It is hardly surprising that there has been an explosion in iatrogenic disease.

There is no easy, slick solution to this massive problem.

But there are some things we can do to restore

some sense to health care and to reduce the appalling incidence of iatrogenic disease.

First, we need to humanise doctors – by stripping away some of their power and authority. Normally assertive and strong individuals who would confront or argue with almost anyone else they might come into contact with often find it difficult to argue with or to confront or question doctors because they have always been encouraged to regard members of the medical profession as 'different'. Doctors are treated with reverence rather than simple respect and that is a terribly unhealthy state of affairs.

In the interests of good health, doctors should throw away all the symbols of authority they currently use – the white coat, and maybe even the title of doctor. And they should certainly get rid of the ubiquitous desk which separates patient from physician.

Next, we need to encourage patients to start treating doctors more critically; to be more demanding, more questioning and more assertive. The evidence shows that assertive patients live longer but I also suspect that assertive patients are less likely to be killed by incompetence. Patients need to be encouraged to take back responsibility for their own health and to learn to regard doctors as technicians – to be consulted but regarded with the scepticism currently reserved for garage mechanics.

We should encourage nurses and other health professionals to be less subservient and more questioning too.

It is surprising how often well trained nurses will

accept absurd and dangerous instructions from inexperienced and ignorant doctors simply because of the traditional subservient position of nurses in relation to doctors.

Third, and perhaps most important of all, we need to make a genuine effort to separate the medical profession from the drug industry. During the last few decades the two have become far too closely intertwined, and today the drug industry dominates the profession; members of the medical establishment are far too uncritical of the industry. It is difficult to see how a group of people who get all their information and instructions from an industry can call themselves a profession. Today, the majority of doctors admit that they never attend any postgraduate education at all. The little that doctors do learn about new treatments comes from the companies promoting their products. It is a bit like airline pilots relying on the company's promotional literature when climbing aboard an aeroplane for the first time. Even Dr Pietroni of St Mary's Hospital Medical School, who helps to educate doctors, admits that 'over forty per cent of the information which influences their decisions as to what to prescribe is received by them directly from drug companies'. We need to encourage doctors to take a more cynical and sceptical look at the claims made by the big drug companies.

Finally, we need to introduce annual tests of doctors. We don't allow old cars onto the roads unless they pass an MOT test. Airline pilots have to undergo regular tests. We should not allow old surgeons into the operating theatre unless they have shown that they have made some effort to keep up to date. Old physicians whose knowledge has passed its sell by date should be forcibly retired.

Doctors have a tremendous position of power and can probably do more harm than any other group of individuals in the community. But once a man or woman receives a degree certificate he or she is given a licence for life. Who would willingly fly in a plane piloted by a man who had passed his exam 50 years earlier and had not made any attempt to keep up to date?

I agree with everything contained in this reprinted article except the last two paragraphs. Having previously demonstrated the ignorance of GPs not only GPs but also medical specialists, who does he think is going to do the instructing and improving? I believe that improvement in medical practice will never be achieved until the present self-satisfaction of the profession is shaken by a tightly argued demonstration of their failures backed up by evidence that points the way of improvement. In other words, they should attend to what I have written in this book about Dr Horrobin, Professor Kennedy and Ivan Illich – advice which applies equally to the statements of Drs Coleman, Gould and Freed. Finally, there is myself.

What effect has the work of these five doctors, one professor of law and one philosopher had on the medical establishment and the overall view of Parliament and the public? Sadly, the answer must be none. The reason for this failure is the absence of a coordinated strategy by us as individuals. Each one of us has had brief bursts of publicity when the papers, radio, and television thought the subject newsworthy, but without a sustained effort such moments pass into relative oblivion. For my own part, I have persevered ever since my six years in Darwen confirmed to me that medical teaching in this century was badly conceived and is responsible for the faults in medical thinking today.

The two subjects with which I am now closely identified are asthma and arthritis. I have made my case quite clear as regards asthma. I have no real quarrel with the establishment on this subject because I have published nothing up to now. In my own defence, though, I would like to make the following statement:

The enormous success of *Arthritis : Is Your Suffering Really Necessary?* in 1981 identified my name in the media as a rheumatologist. As John Hale had told me, such a success would ensure interest and attention in any other subject about which I chose to write. I respected his views and now know that he was right.

However, I remained very worried about the lot of asthmatics. I therefore phoned the Asthma Research Council and spoke to a consultant there – I think his name was Dr Smith. I asked him if he had any idea at all what the underlying cause of the increase in numbers and severity of the disease was, together with the increased death rate. He quite readily said no. I then explained to him my views on the problem and illustrated it with two cases. He was manifestly interested in my argument and suggested I write a paper on it and send it to the *British Medical Journal* and the *Lancet*. I told him that my experience of these journals led me to believe that it would not be printed, but I would think about it.

I realized that the success of my book was with the media and the public, not with the profession. If, at that time, I were to write an article on asthma, it might very well be seized upon by the profession as evidence that my thirst for publicity had led me to present myself as a specialist not only in rheumatology but in asthma as well. What a field day they would have hunting down this Fox! So, I finally decided not to write, then hoped the success of that book would allow me to publish *Asthma: Is Your Suffering Really Necessary?* very much sooner than has been the case. What transpired since then is the true story of the dismissal of my book and treatment by a Dr Dudley Hart, a leading member of the Arthritis and Rheumatism Council. Only he can account for his behaviour, although I can make some intelligent guesses.

The story starts with almost the last of the very many press reviews, television and radio broadcasts aired after the publication of my book in August 1981. It was on Radio 4's *Does He Take Sugar?*, a programme aimed specifically at people with a disability, some time around the end of April 1982. Shortly afterwards a patient asked me if I had heard the same station broadcast a 'response' on 13 May 1982. 'No,' I replied. He then told me that a Dr Hart had been making silly and derogatory remarks about my work. I contacted Radio 4 and soon they sent me a transcript of the recording, of which this is an extract:

MULHERN   Mrs Lee Baker of Dudley, West Midlands and Mrs E. Forester of Ivybridge, Devon, both write in to complain that they can't convince their general practitioners of the value of Dr W. Fox's book on arthritis. Why do the experts tend to ignore him, they ask? Well Dr Hart, what was Dr W. Fox all about?

HART   Well Dr Fox thought that allergy came into it and then if you used certain anti-allergic drugs these would help. Well, really there's no evidence of that at all. Second thing he says, that he can spot and early rheumatoid by ... coming up ... by injecting certain areas, in their fingers for instance, and they'll swear ... with aspirin funnily enough ... and that he can nip it in the bud by so doing. Aspirin, you see, has been used since 1899 in big enough doses to saturate not only the little fingers but the whole body and so all he's doing really is putting aspirin to a small area, one area ... one part ... and he claims that he can detect where the arthritis starts and nip it in the bud there. Now I don't know if this has been repeated by anybody else because it is the most difficult thing in the world to find a rheumatoid at that very early stage, so I think the answer to your question is that none of us see rheumatoids that early and we would need much more evidence than has already been put up before it's really worth looking into.

What he says about allergy must be seen in its correct context. It comprises only one factor out of eight listed and dealt with in the book. In spite of what he said I can assure my readers that it is a very valuable adjunct to the treatment of those patients who have an identifiable allergic factor in their history. However it is not important enough to engage in a serious discussion of my work. Because the remainder of his reply bears no relation to what I have written. I expressed the view that he could not have read the book and this he never denied. It is therefore essential that I give you a clear résumé of what is actually in the book. The 'treatment' which he describes in a totally incoherent manner is actually presented by me as clinical evidence in support of my thesis that arthritis does not start in the joints but as an inflammation in the superficial connective tissue related to the joints and can be a considerable distance from them. These areas I call rheumatic patches and where they are injected with the aspirin solution (it is really sodium salicylate a salt of aspirin, a word which everybody knows and can remember) a most remarkable result ensues within one or two minutes. The pain and stiffness around the joint is either eliminated or so markedly reduced that there follows a spectacular improvement in the functioning of the affected joint.

At this point the immediate result is all that is needed to support my claim that there are rheumatic patches in the superficial connective tissue and that they are directly related to the joint dysfunction. The improvement can last but a few minutes in some cases and up to several days and weeks in others and these differences are fully discussed in the text. What is really important is that I have demonstrated a method and a mechanism which no known form of treatment can even approach. This procedure can be successfully repeated in any part of the body and in any number of cases. Countless thousands of these treatments have been given by myself and many other doctors who have read my books and have attended my clinics. Over the ensuing years further study and experience has increased my understanding of the problem whilst improvement in techniques has produced better and more lasting results. I am fully aware that this discovery challenges the very basis of the orthodox thinking and practice in arthritis treatment. I have accepted this formidable task because I can still recall the shock I experienced when I realized that all my years of clinical research had led me to test my theory with the aspirin solution and the results were way beyond what I had dared to hope.

It took me a long time and many repetitions of the experiment before I could actually believe it was true. So, I do understand why doctors' first reaction would be disbelief and opposition to ideas which challenge their thinking and treatment. However I cannot find the slightest tolerance for the 'views' of those who oppose my case without making some effort to understand this new concept in a field of medicine where failure is the only word which describes fifty years of research and practice.

As if providence intervened, a few days later an official from the Civil Service Stores in Westminster telephoned to ask if I could supply a copy of my book as it was urgently required by one of its customers. The book had been selling so fast that the printer had been unable to keep up with the demand. During this conversation I discovered that their customer was Dr F. Dudley Hart, the very same person who made the broadcast you have read. Of course, I had already sent a written complaint to the BBC. As you will see, he had been informed about it, and was thus anxious to read the book, which I arranged to be sent to him.

At this point, I clearly had excellent grounds for a claim for damages. However, I was not interested in material gains – only in a fair hearing for my researches and results. It was the welfare of millions of sufferers that I cared about.

Judge for yourself the correspondence between Dr Hart and myself, which is reprinted in chronological order. It is followed by one relevant communication with the BBC.

19th July, 1982

Dear Dr Dudley Hart,

I am writing about your broadcast on May 13th, a transcript of which I believe you have.

I was very sad to hear how you referred to my work. It was all too obvious that you could not have read either of my books.

Many doctors and some rheumatologists have seen demonstration of my methods and not a single one has failed to be impressed.

May I suggest that you spare the time to come to my home where I have patients every day except Wednesday.

You can then see the treatment in operation and you will be quite free to talk to the patients. I look forward to hearing from you.

Yours sincerely,

28th July, 1982

Dear Dr Fox,

Many thanks for your letter. It is very kind of you to invite me to your home. I am, however, only just back from holiday, and am trying to catch up with a back-log of appointments, but I would be pleased to visit you some time later. In the meantime, I wonder if you would send me a copy of your book together with the bill, for I would be glad to have my own copy. Could you do this.

With all good wishes.

Yours sincerely,

1st August, 1982

Dear Dr Dudley Hart,

Enclosed please find book as requested and the account.

There is an earlier book (1975) *Arthritis & Allied Conditions – A New & Successful Approach* (£5), which I can let you have if you wish.

It was the refusal of rheumatologists to review this earlier book which obliged me to write the second one. The enormous success of this book has given rise to a paperback edition which is due out in late September.

I am particularly anxious that you should be aware of the reality that my clinical findings and treatment represent a positive and decisive step forward in the understanding of these diseases.

Writing and reading can never be as convincing as an actual demonstration. Would you please make an effort to see this as early as possible? Your support, if you were as satisfied with the demonstration as other doctors have been, would be invaluable.

Kind regards.

Very sincerely,

[Undated compliment slip]
Many thanks for the speedy delivery. I will come back to you later re visit and your earlier book also.

22nd August, 1982

Dear Dr Hart,

I wonder if you would give me a date when we will be able to meet. My time is rapidly being taken up in demonstrating and teaching, and I do want to reserve a date for you.

As I indicated in a previous letter, I am very anxious for your support – if you are satisfied with the demonstration. I would prefer this before the paperback edition of my book appears on September 30th next.

Kind regards.

Yours sincerely,

21st October 1982

Dear Marlene Pease [editor of BBC Radio 4's *Does He Take Sugar?*],

Re: Dr Dudley Hart & myself

Since I have received the transcript I contacted Dr Hart and this is a chronicle of events since:

1. *19th July*. I sent the letter copy enclosed.
2. *28th July*. His reply in which he asked for a copy of my book and expressed a desire to visit me after he had completed a backlog of patients.
3. *1st Aug*. My letter, copy enclosed.
4. *3rd Aug*. His reply, acknowledgment and promise to contact me later.
5. *22nd Aug*. My letter. Up to date no reply.

I think you must agree I have been very patient. I see no excuse for his failure to implement his promise.

I hope you will now agree that I should be given a right of reply at an early date – it is 5 months since the broadcast.

Yours sincerely,

The outcome of these negotiations was that the BBC gave me another broadcast but made no mention of Dr Hart. So the public was never told about his condemnation of a book he had never read and a treatment he did not understand. I accepted this result philosophically, as another example of the difficulty in fighting the establishment – in this case not only Dr Hart, as a member of the Arthritis and Rheumatism Council, but also the BBC, keen to evade their partial responsibility for the broadcast.

Years went by; I lectured and demonstrated my work whenever I had the opportunity. Then came the sequel to the story of Dr Hart and the BBC.

In November 1990 my third book (co-authored with Dr J.L. Freed) was published by Macmillan: *Understanding Arthritis*. In January 1991 Radio 4 invited me to be interviewed for *Does He Take Sugar?* I accepted and, at their request, took along a patient on 17 January. The interview was duly recorded and they said it would be broadcast in about two to three weeks. It was eventually transmitted on 24 March. I listened to it and was horrified when the same Dr Hart was now given an immediate opportunity to criticize the book and the recording. The BBC had failed to inform me and had given me no opportunity for a right of reply. Here is the transcript in full:

SPEAKER: What he calls the rheumatic patch. His hypothesis is based on his findings among hundreds of patients at the Chart House Rheumatism Clinic in the Orthopaedic Department of the Royal Homoeopathic Hospital and in general practice. I asked Dr Fox how he treats people with arthritis.

FOX: I have now been able to demonstrate that the disease does not start in the joints and it doesn't matter whether it is rheumatoid or osteo-arthritis. The disease starts in the connective tissue. This is a tissue which is vital to any form of walking.

SPEAKER: So if it starts in the connective tissue how are you then able to treat it?

FOX: By injecting the appropriate rheumatic patches as I have called them with a very weak solution of sodium salicylate. In fact one treatment uses the equivalent of one third of one aspirin tablet and that's all the patient on the average requires once a week in the first stages of treatment.

SPEAKER: And how much success have you seen with this treatment?

FOX: I have always claimed round about 80 per cent. I may say that my treatment has been adopted in Bulgaria. It was so successful there that they have established treatment in every district hopsital in Bulgaria.

SPEAKER: Well, Connie Blake, you've been treated through this method. First of all perhaps you can tell me how severe your condition was.

CONNIE BLAKE: I had a lot of pain in my back, hips and knees for many years and at that time my hands were extremely painful, red and swollen and I had lost my grip and worst of all my wrists were actually locking. I was told that all that could be done for me was to increase the dose of the drug

Brufen which I was taking, give me a jacket for my spine and fuse my wrists. I was horrified at these suggestions. I previously heard quite by chance Dr Fox being interviewed on Radio. I saw Dr Fox in November 1981 and upon examination he told me I was full of arthritis. However, Dr injected above my wrists and immediately my fingers and wrists felt as though they had been oiled. The inflammation subsided, I had a good grip again and my wrists have never locked since.

SPEAKER: Dr Fox, does it stand alone as the treatment or does it have to be supplemented by other drugs?

FOX: The only other treatment in the form of drugs is an anti-histamine which I generally advise most patients to take regularly.

SPEAKER: What about non-drug treatment because a lot of people recommend exercise and diet as a way of helping off?

FOX: This is all. Exercise does not improve it – it makes it worse.

SPEAKER: I understand that sodium salicylate is basically a form of aspirin which has been tried but very often discounted as a treatment by other arthritis specialists. Why, if this is all it is, is it necessary to inject it? Wouldn't it be more comfortable and more convenient to take it orally?

FOX: What I am doing is injecting the aspirin at the point where the inflammation is and that gives immediate relief within a minute or two and in order to get an aspirin effect on that the patients would need to take so much aspirin it would be impossible for them to take it without great damage.

SPEAKER: Well I then put some of those points to Dr Frank Dudley Hart of the Arthritis and Rheumatism Council.

HART: Well he's right in as much as most of these arthropathies are started and very often by infection and then spread throughout the body and affect the joints and things later on but the idea of it all starting in the superficial connective tissue there is no evidence of this at all and just by injecting certain parts of the superficial connective tissue really doesn't make any difference. It is also untrue to say that all arthropathies are connected in this way because osteo-arthritis, the commonest of the lot, is partly inflammatory but mostly wear and tear and really the connective tissue only comes in there as a very secondary thing.

SPEAKER: But it's claimed that the treatment is 80 per cent effective.

HART: Well if you look at the book, it's improvement – it's not cure. It's improvement and of course all sorts of treatment acupuncture all sorts of things you get a 70–80 per cent improvement for the time being. But there is no evidence that it seems to switch anything off. Which is the

SPEAKER: big hope that this sort of treatment might. So this immediate relief which he talks about within a couple of minutes of the injection is simply a temporary measure?

HART: It's a temporary measure, yes, what you get immediately with sodium salicylate is – it isn't aspirin, by the way, it's sodium salicylate – is an intense pain where you have the injection that hurts like old Harry for a bit and then he points out that he would rather have that than give the procaine which means two injections and this is followed by temporary ease which may last several days or longer but it doesn't last forever.

SPEAKER: Isn't the treatment, though, a tried and tested method – sodium salicylate?

HART: Oh, sodium salicylate, yes, it was the treatment for old rheumatic fever, for instance, and it was taken by mouth in biggish doses as he says. But no firm put it out for injection. It isn't available under the National Health or in any of the pharmacopoeial books as a solution to inject.

SPEAKER: But isn't anything worth a try with something so chronic and painful as arthritis?

HART: Oh yes, oh yes, I think so. I think anything is worth a try but it has to be … we have so many of these things put up to us – it has to make some sort of sense, really, and I know that in many of these cases anyway the patients have gone to other doctors later – that it hasn't had any lasting effect. This temporary effect is all you get and there is nothing to show, really, so far on the evidence that he produces that it aborts or negatives anything.

SPEAKER: So what's your advice then?

HART: I would think on evidence that although he gets results with this as you do with any form of injection these injections do produce relief but they don't produce a cure.

SPEAKER: Dr Frank Dudley Hart.

I then went back to the BBC with my complaint. After many fruitless attempts to get some action from Colin Hughes, the producer of the programme, I finally wrote the following letter to Michael Green, the controller of Radio 4.

12th June, 1991

Dear Mr Green,
Re: *DOES HE TAKE SUGAR?*

Following the publication of my latest book *Understanding Arthritis*, I was invited to speak on this programme. The interview was recorded on 17th January and, after many changes of date, was broadcast on 24th March.

When I heard it I realised the cause of the delay – they had to wait on Dr Dudley Hart. At no time did they indicate to me that he, or anybody else, was to record his views on what I had said, or presumably what he had read in my book.

Furthermore, they omitted my answer to the

question about trials posed by the interviewer. This answer showed that there was a great interest in the work I was doing, by many responsible members of the rheumatology discipline.

Dr Hart's statement contained, amongst others, the following remark which is absolutely untrue: Quote Oh sodium salicylate yes it was the treatment for old rheumatic fever for instance and it was taken by mouth in biggish doses as he says. But no firm put it out for injection it isn't available under the National Health Unquote. It has been manufactured by McCarthy for over 20 years and it is prescribable on the NHS. It is also used by a number of GPs and specialists.

Much else of what he said is nebulous, misleading and irrelevant. In 1982 he answered questions about my work on this same programme which followed two weeks after a broadcast by me relating to my previous book *Arthritis: Is Your Suffering Really Necessary?*

He did not disclose then that he had not read my book and made the foolish remarks about my work to sufferers who wanted to know why they couldn't get my treatment locally.

I have all the evidence that I supplied him with a copy of my book, for which he paid, and his assurance that he would accept my invitation to attend a clinic where he could see for himself the actual treatment and its results. This very friendly settlement was reached through my personal intervention. I was not interested in litigation or damages, my concern is purely for the unnecessary suffering of patients. He never kept his promise to contact me.

The BBC, however, did make amends by giving me a second interview when I was able to put the record straight.

I think you must agree that the choice of Dr Dudley Hart, without telling me, was extremely unfortunate.

After hearing the broadcast, I 'phoned Colin Hughes and complained. I asked for a tape of the interview to be expedited – it was promised at the recording session. I waited for about 3 weeks – nothing happened. I then 'phoned Colin Hughes again. He was not available but his assistant offered to take down my complaints and would ensure that they were discussed, and that I would receive the tape together with an answer to my queries. Again nothing happened.

I then decided to make a personal approach to Dr Dudley Hart. I spoke to him on the 'phone, he was busy with a patient, could not spare the time to talk with me, and was not prepared to give an alternative convenient time. He claimed he was entitled to his opinion.

Well, I have done all I can to resolve this highly unsatisfactory state of affairs.

As I have indicated, there are many other criticisms of his statements which can be challenged, but I have tried to keep this letter as short as possible and sufficiently factual, so that you can realise that what I am seeking is that the truth of what I write in my books shall not be blemished by untruths from a doctor in so influential a position as he holds.

Personalities should be irrelevant to scientific progress. Seeking and speaking the truth is what the BBC stands for and what the public, in particular the millions of rheumatic suffers, have a right to expect.

I would like this problem to be resolved as quickly and sensibly as possible and look forward to hearing from you.

Yours sincerely,

This brought no reply at all. I then phoned the BBC and after much to-ing and fro-ing I was connected to a Caroline Millington. She made some excuses for the absence of a reply and promised some action. After further delay, I was told that Marlene Pease, editor of *Does He Take Sugar?* would be coming to see me. She came in late August and stayed for something like two hours. We had a thorough discussion in the most friendly and understanding way, which she later followed up with this letter.

4th September 1991

Dear Dr Fox,

I very much enjoyed our meeting last week and as a result of our conversation have asked reporter James Whitbourn to make a feature with and about you for DOES HE TAKE SUGAR?

We want to look at the struggle you have had as a GP to try and get your treatment for arthritis recognized, and the particular problems GPs incur in trying to set up controlled clinical trials, opposition from consultants, and the general convervatism of the medical fraternity. I understand there has been a recent change in the law regarding the indemnity of doctors and we shall be seeking clarification of this from the Department of Health and the British Medical Association.

I have already been in touch with the Westminster Hospital who will contribute to the piece and I made careful notes on all the other contacts you gave me. If you can make contact with the girl you think might have been having treatment for a period of ten years, I would be grateful.

Yours sincerely,

The Westminster Hospital was the fourth British hospital that had attempted to start double blind trials of my work. They had already initiated open trials. Eventually the BBC broadcast a programme, which dealt with some of my struggles very satisfactorily, but spent too much time on the research problems of a Dr Cox. These issues were mostly irrelevant to my core concerns. In the run-up to the broadcast, I experienced again the aloofness of the medical establishment.

Marlene Pease told me that Dr Cox, a member of the executive of the Royal College of General Practitioners, was taking part in the programme. Always on the alert for a possible ally – after all I started life as a GP – I called the Royal College. I explained why I wanted to speak to him personally (nowadays you always have to do that before you can speak to any doctor). The secretary told me he would be there in two days' time but if I tried his surgery in Birmingham, I might catch him. She gave me the number and I phoned immediately.

I spoke to the receptionist, who said he was not on duty that evening. 'Well, could you give me a number where I could contact him?' No, she could not do that, but if I explained the reason I wanted to contact him, she would try to pass on the message. I told her the story of the imminent broadcast – it was the next day – and why I would like to have a word with him. She seemed quite impressed, took my number and said she would contact Dr Cox immediately. I felt sure he would soon ring me back.

Not a word came from him – neither that evening nor the next day when he actually received another message at the Royal College in London. It doesn't take long for the delusion of self-importance to spread from consultant to GP! Of course, if Dr Cox had not been so snooty about my approach to him, I might have acquired the backing of the Royal College of General Practitioners.

Ultimately, I was fobbed off a second time in my efforts to be given the right of reply to Dr Hart's views as a member of the Arthritis Research Council. On this occasion, the programme was broadcast some fifteen months after my complaint. In fairness to Marlene Pease, the editor, I would say that the programme was excellent in the way it dealt with my work and my problems, but absolutely no mention was made of Dr Hart's behaviour.

Imagine the difference it would have made if he had taken the view that Dr Charles MacWorth Young took when he read my book, or indeed other consultants like Professor Maini of the Kennedy Instiute, where he invited me to lecture. Dr Jan Wojtulewski of the Eastbourne General Hospital would also have given my theories a quite different press. At his outpatients departments I was able to demonstrate my work on five consecutive Wednesdays, with quite remarkable results.

If the present trials of my arthritis treatment had been started some twelve or thirteen years ago, I would long ago have been free to write this book on asthma. I could not do it before, because I would have left myself open to charges of claiming to be a specialist in two entirely different subjects. This is pure anathema to medical thinking, which over the years has developed so many specializations you would think that only by subdividing a living human being could you hope to solve all of their problems.

I have dealt with this matter at some length because it demonstrates how difficult it is to break the resistance of the medical establishment. The BBC is rather different, having always taken an interest in what I have had to say. I was greatly supported by all BBC television and radio stations when in 1981–2 my book on arthritis was published.

I understand their difficulty. They suffer from the same inhibitions as most medical and scientific correspondents of the press, who find it difficult to believe that the medical fraternity are not all lily-white.

Unfortunately, having retired I can no longer undertake to treat patients on a large scale. I am, however, willing to treat a small group of about five or six, if their GPs would be prepared to co-operate in the trial. Ideally a group practice in North London, where I live, would be most suitable. I also know that Dr L.J. Freed would be prepared to do an even more extensive trial in Manchester.

When one considers the uncountable billions that have been spent in research on arthritis during the last sixty to seventy years in all the countries of the world, is it not remarkable that we are no nearer to a solution of this problem than we were at the outset? And yet we continue to pour our resources down this endless drain. On the way, we have submitted countless animals to unnatural and tortured lives and countless patients to immeasurable drug treatments that have led to suffering on a grand scale and sometimes death.

The situation of asthma, which has been with us for only twenty-five years, is exactly parallel, and if research continues on the same lines, we will reach the same impasse in another twenty-five years. The tragedy is that, apart from the colossal cost, the human suffering will continue, whilst the deaths will increase to maybe five or six thousand per year. What other branch of human activity would tolerate such expense and failure? Indeed other branches of science and technology would long ago have discarded such methods, realizing there must be faultlines that need to be uncovered.

One can only hope that a widespread airing of the facts and logic of the argument will sooner or later have its effect on the participants – be they doctors, scientists, technological staff or patients – to cry, 'Stop. What are we doing so wrongly?' Well, everybody, who has read my books should have more than an inkling of the answer:

Medical researchers are applying scientific methods to a problem that they have not conceived in the right way. If you are confronted by an algebraic equation, say

$$\frac{x-y}{z} = z-m+h$$

you will never be able to solve it by using other branches of mathematics such as trigonometry or calculus. You must first worry about the problem in its own terms, algebra. Only then will you have an idea how to proceed to an understanding. The problem in both arthritis and asthma is exactly the same. They are using pharmacology – a very incomplete science – to treat two diseases whose very onset they do not understand, much less their whole natural histories or possible causes. This explains why early contributors to the thoughts in this book are right to blame the medical profession for not only failing to understand problems but actually causing needless suffering and sometimes death.

In the case of asthma – now an acute problem – it should be relatively simple for doctors to follow my advice and see the relatively rapid decline in the severity of the disease and the number of deaths even in one year. Perhaps this is the ideal opportunity for the Royal College of General Practitioners to claim that clinical research into disease should be returned to or, at least, shared with GPs, who live and work amongst patients. This would achieve some sort of balance between specialists, who know so much about their subjects (and thus tend to have closed minds), and doctors in general practice, who have gleaned so little from so much (and thus might have more open minds). Some GPs will surely be able to contribute views and ideas that they have accumulated by observation and examination of their patients before, during, and after a diagnosis and treatment was made.

Finally let me state quite clearly that nowhere in my papers or books have I ever claimed to cure any disease. What I have done is to erect signposts in the clinical study of various diseases, which I hope will indicate a more fruitful line of enquiry towards the understanding of those diseases. There are four which I have used in this book:

1. Improved teaching of clinical medicine
2. The distinction between illness and disease
3. The rheumatic patch in arthritis
4. Ignorance and fear in asthma

When these signposts are read and understood we can begin to solve the medical problems that afflict increasing millions of patients across this century. Only then can the words of our professor of medicine, enunciated at our first lecture come true. 'When you qualify as a doctor you will become a member of the most noble profession in the world, because we are dedicated to our own extinction by the elimination of disease.'

Judging by the enormous increase in the cost of health care (about £40 billion per year), we appear to be travelling in the wrong direction.

I hope in the course of this book you will have gained a real understanding of the true nature and history of asthma and how simply it can be managed. This is the knowledge to which every patient has the right to have access, a principle that has dominated my thinking and researches.

Unlike medical scientists, my laboratory has been the consulting room, my tools have been an open mind, a willingness to listen and believe what patients tell me, followed by a detailed examination of the body and finally explaining my conclusion to the patient. I trust you find yourself in accord with this presentation of the asthma problem. If it has given you some hope then you, the reader, should take responsibility for demanding more co-operation from the medical profession. Once a number of doctors have begun to see the madness of present-day treatment of asthma, they will very soon realize that I have never been attacking *them*, but the method of teaching in medical schools and hospitals to which they have been subjected.

Wouldn't it be wonderful if asthma was returned to its state prior to antibiotics – no hospitalization, no drugs, no deaths: just a nuisance which can be eradicated quite easily. When this is achieved, we must make sure that the £2 billion is not then wasted on other futile treatment, or squandered on some research establishment that claims their discovery of a new gene is 'world shattering'. Such developments represent only a tiny facet of the truly awesome creation of the living body and mind.

It is only this realization that can hope to instil humility, such a vital ingredient for every scientist and doctor. Nature can never be beaten: one must learn to understand, respect and work with her. The uncritical and uncontrolled use of drugs is the very antithesis of this concept and can never succeed.

References

1. Serafini, U.: 'Can fatal asthma be prevented? – A personal view'. *Clin. Exp. Allergy* 1992, *22*: 576–588.
2. Osler, W.: *The Principles and Practice of Medicine*, p. 500 (Young J. Pentland, Edinburgh, 1892).
3. Christian, H.A. & Mackenzie, J. (eds) *The Oxford Medicine*, p. 232 (OUP, 1920).
4. Coke, F.: *Asthma*, p. 104 (Wright & Sons, Bristol, 1923).
5. Conybeare, J.J.: *A Textbook of Medicine*, p. 486 (Livingstone, Edinburgh, 1929).
6. Burney, P.G.J.: *Strategy for Asthma, BMJ,* 1991, *303*: 571–3.
7. Sears, M.R.: 'Epidemiology of asthma', in Flenley, D.C., Petty, T.L. (eds) *Recent Advances in Respiratory Medicine* vol. 4, 1–11 (Churchill Livingstone, Edinburgh, 1986).
8. Haahtela, I., Lindholm, H., Bjorksten, F., Koskenvuo, K. & Laitinen, L.: 'Prevalence of Asthma in Finnish Young Men', *B.M.J.,* 1990, *301*: 266–8.
9. Burney, P.G.J., Chinn, S. & Rona, R.J.: 'Has the prevalence of asthma increased in children? Evidence from the national study of health and growth, *BMJ,* 1990, *300*: 1306–10.
10. Sheffer, A.L., quoted by B. Zweiman in open letter to members of the American Academy of Allergy & Immunology, July 1991.
11. Crane, J., Pearce, N. Beasley, R. & Burgess, C.: 'Worldwide worsening wheezing – is the cure the cause?, *Lancet* 1992, *339*: 814.
12. Khot, A. & Burn, R.: Deaths from Asthma, *BMJ,* 1984, *289*: 557.
13. Sly, R.M.: Increases in deaths from asthma, *Ann Allergy* 1984, *53*: 20–25.
14. Mullaly, D.I., Howard W.A., Hubbard, T.J., Grauman, J.S. & Cohen, S.G.: 'Increased hospitalizations for asthma among children in the Washington DC area during 1961–1981, *Ann Allergy* 1984, *53*: 15–19.
15. Shaw, R.A., Crane, J. & O'Donnell, T.V.: Prevalence of asthma in children, *BMJ,* 1990, *300*: 1652–3.

16. Robertson, C.F., Heycock, E., Bishop, J., Nolan, T., Olinsky, A. & Phelan, P.D.: 'Prevalence of asthma in Melbourne school-children: changes over 26 years, *BMJ*, 1991, *303*: 1116–8.

17. Sheffer, A.L.: International Consensus Report on Diagnosis and Treatment of Asthma, *Clin. Exp. Allergy* 1992, *22 suppl 1*: xi.

18. Godlee, F.: Air pollution I – from pea souper to photochemical smog, *BMJ*, 1991, *303*: 1459–61.

19. Editorial: Asthma and the bean, *Lancet*, 1989, *ii*: 538–40.

20. Sporik, R., Holgate, S.T., Platts-Mills, T.A.E., Cogswell, J.J.: 'Exposure to house dust mite allergen (Der pI) and the development of asthma in childhood – a prospective study, *New Engl. J. Med.*, 1990, *323*: 502–7.

21. Pattemore, P.K., Johnston S.L. & Bardin P.G.: 'Viruses as precipitants of asthma symptoms I, Epidemiology'. *Clin. Exp. Allergy* 1992, 22: 325–336.

22. Rees, J.: Beta-2 agonists and asthma (editorial, *BMJ*, 1991, *302*: 1166–7.

23. Elwood, J.M.: Fenoterol and fatal asthma, *Lancet*, 1990, **336**: 436–7.

24. Rees, H.A., Millar, J.S. & Donald, K.W.: Adrenaline in bronchial asthma, *Lancet*, 1967, *ii*: 1164–7.

25. Rees, H.A., Borthwick, R.C., Millar, J.S. & Donald, K.W.: 'Aminophylline in bronchial asthma', *ibid* 1167–9.

26. Toennesen, J., Lowry, R. & Lambert, P.M.: 'Oral theophylline and fatal asthma, *Lancet*, 1981, *ii*: 200–1.

27. Sears, M.R.: Beta-2 agonists and asthma, *BMJ*, 1991, *303*: 123.

28. Vathenen, A.S., Knox, A.J., Higgins, B.G., Britton, J.R. & Tattersfield A.E.: 'Rebound increase in bronchial responsiveness after treatment with inhaled terbutaline', *Lancet*, 1988, *i*: 554–8.

29. Rolla, G. & Bucca, C.: 'Magnesium, beta-agonists and asthma, *Lancet*, 1988, *i*: 989.

30. Sears, M.R.: Dose reduction of beta-agonists in asthma, *Lancet* 1991, *338*: 1331–2.

31. van Schayck, C.P., Dompeling, E., van Herwaarden, C.L.A., Folgering, H., Verbeek A.L.M., van der Hoogen H.J.M., van Weel, C.: 'Bronchodilator treatment in moderate asthma or chronic bronchitis: Continuous or on demand? A randomised controlled study', *BMJ*, 1991, *303*: 1426–31.

32. Godlee, F. & Walker, A.: 'Importance of a healthy environment', *BMJ*, 1991, *303*: 1124–6.

33. Robinson, R.: 'Wheezy children', *BMJ*, 1991, *302*: 1516.

34. Reid, L.M.: 'The presence or absence of bronchial mucus in fatal asthma, '*J. Allergy Clin. Immunol* 1987, *80*: 415–6.

35. Hogg, J.C., Hulbert, W.C., Armour, C. & Pare, P.D.: 'The effect

of mucosal inflammation in airways reactivity', *in* Kay, A.B., Austen, K.F. & Lichtenstein, L.M. (eds) *Asthma: Physiology, Immunopharmacology, and Treatment*, Academic Press, London, 1984, 327–38.

36. Freed, D.L.J.: 'The immunology of allergy', *in* Rees, A.J. & Purcell, H. (eds) *Disease and the Environment*, Wiley, London, 1982, pp. 65–78.

37. Horsfield, K. (1981), cited by Buckley, C.J.: 'The role of bronchial musculature', *Lancet* 1989, *ii*: 836–7.

38. Capewell, S., Reynolds, S., Shuttleworth, D., Edwards, C. & Finlay, A.Y.: 'Purpura and dermal thinning associated with high dose inhaled steroids', *BMJ*, 1990, *300*: 1548–51.

39. Corrigan, C.: 'Mechanism of glucocorticoid action in asthma; too little, too late', *Clin Exp Allergy* 1992, *22*: 315–7.

40. Freed, D.L.J., Buckley, C.H.: 'Mucotractive effect of lectin', *Lancet* 1978, *i*: 585–6.

41. Freed, D.L.J.: 'Lectins in food: their importance in health and disease'. *J Nutr Med* 1991, *2*: 45–64.

42. Brompton Hospital/MRC Collaborative Committee: Long term study of disodium chromoglycate in treatment of severe extrinsic or intrinsic bronchial asthma in adults, *BMJ*, 1972, *4*: 383–8.

43. Freed, D.L.J., Buckley, C.H., Tsivion, Y., Sharon, N. & Katz, D.H.: 'Non-allergenic haemolysins in grass pollens and housedust mites', *Allergy*, 1983, *38*: 477–486.

44. Dudgeon, D.L., Parker, F.B. Fritelli, G. & Rabuzzi, D.D.: 'Bronchiectasis in pediatric patients resulting from aspirated grass inflorescences'. *Arch Surg*, 1980, *115*: 979–983.

45. Heino, M., Monkare, S., Haahtela, T. & Laitinen, L.A.: 'An electron-microscopic study of the airways in patients with farmer's lung', *Eur J Respir Dis*, 1982, *63*: 52–61.

46. Seely, S., Freed, D.L.J., Silverstone, G. & Rippere, V.: *Diet-Related Diseases The Modern Epidemic*, Croom Helm, London, 1985.

47. Fox, W.W.: personal communication.

48. Kalra, S., Owen, S.J., Hepworth, J. & Woodcock, A.: 'Airborne house dust antigen after vacuum cleaning', *Lancet* 1990, *336*: 449.

49. Arshad, S.H., Matthews, S., Gant, C. & Hide, D.W.: 'Effect of allergen avoidance on development of allergic disorders in infancy', *Lancet* 1992, *339*: 1493–97.

50. Jarrett, E.E.: 'Perinatal influences on IgE responses', *Lancet* 1984, *ii*: 797–9.

51. Roberts, S.A. & Soothill, J.F.: 'Provocation of allergic response by supplementary feeds of cow's milk', *Arch Dis Child* 1982, *57*: 127–30.

52. Morrow Brown, H.: 'Milk allergy and intolerance: clinical

aspects', *in* Freed, D.L.J. (ed), *Health Hazards of Milk*, Eastbourne, Bailliere Tindall, 1984, p. 103.

53. Ishii, A., Yatani, T., Kato, H. & Fujimoto, T.: 'Mite fauna, housedust and Kawasaki disease', *Lancet*, 1983, *ii*: 102–3.

54. Miller, J.: Personal communication.

Works Mentioned

Fox, William W., *Arthritis & Allied Conditions: A New & Successful Approach*, 1975. [Out of print. Copies available only in public & medical libraries.]

Fox, William W., Arthritis: *Is Your Suffering Really Necessary?* [Out of print. Available only in public libraries.]

Fox, William W. & Freed, D.L.J., *Understanding Arthritis* (Macmillan Press Scientific & Medical, 1990).

European Medical Journal, English edition No. 4, Dr Vernon Coleman, Lynmouth, Devon EX35 SEE. Fax: 0271 882235.

'Asthma Data Mar Pollution Theory', 'Hospital Doctor', p.2, Oct, 1994.